The Jessie and John Danz Lectures

Environmental Health Risks and Public Policy

Decision Making in Free Societies

David V. Bates

UNIVERSITY OF WASHINGTON PRESS

Seattle and London

Copyright © 1994 by the University of Washington Press
Printed in the United States of America

Published simultaneously in Canada by
UBC Press, 6344 Memorial Road,
Vancouver, B.C. Canada V6T 1W5

Library of Congress Cataloging-in-Publication Data

Environmental health risks and public policy : decision making in
free societies / David V. Bates.
    p. cm. — (The Jessie and John Danz lecture series)
  Includes bibliographical references and index.
  ISBN 0–295–97336–6 (cloth : acid-free paper), — ISBN
0–295–97337–4 (paper : acid-free paper)
  1. Environmental health—Government policy—Canada—Decision
making.   2. Environmental health—Government policy—United States—
Decision making.   3. Environmental health—Government policy—Great
Britain—Decision making.   4. Health risk assessment—Canada.
5. Health risk assessment—United States.   6. Health risk
assessment—Great Britain.   I. Title.   II. Series.
RA566.B38   1994   94–2410
363.73—dc20   CIP

The paper used in this publication meets the minimum requirements
of American National Standard for Information Sciences—
Permanence of Paper for Printed Library Materials,
ANSI Z39.48-1984.

The Jessie and John Danz Lectures

I N OCTOBER 1961, Mr. John Danz, a Seattle pioneer, and his wife, Jessie Danz, made a substantial gift to the University of Washington to establish a perpetual fund to provide income to be used to bring to the University of Washington each year "distinguished scholars of national and international reputation who have concerned themselves with the impact of science and philosophy on man's perception of a rational universe." The fund established by Mr. and Mrs. Danz is now known as the Jessie and John Danz Fund, and the scholars brought to the University under its provisions are known as Jessie and John Danz Lecturers or Professors.

Mr. Danz wisely left to the Board of Regents of the University of Washington the identification of the special fields in science, philosophy, and other disciplines in which lectureships may be established. His major concern and interest were that the fund would enable the University of Washington to bring to the campus some of the truly great scholars and thinkers of the world.

Mr. Danz authorized the Regents to expend a portion of the income from the fund to purchase special collections of books, documents, and other scholarly materials needed to reinforce the effectiveness of the extraordinary lectureships and professorships. The terms of the gift also provided for the publication and dissemination, when this seems appropriate, of the lectures given by the Jessie and John Danz Lecturers.

Through this book, therefore, another Jessie and John Danz Lecturer speaks to the people and scholars of the world, as he has spoken to his audiences at the University of Washington and in the Pacific Northwest community.

Contents

Figures

Acknowledgments

I wish to begin by thanking the University of Washington for the honor of the invitation to give the 1993 Jessie and John Danz Lectures on which this book is based. The Danz Lectures are concerned with "the impact of science and philosophy on man's perception of a rational universe." The notes sent to me by the university record details of John Danz's remarkable achievements and of his generous endowment. It is stated that he was an independent and often unorthodox thinker, with deep faith and convictions though a member of no established church, neither a cynic nor an iconoclast, but nevertheless an idealist.

As a Unitarian and a former dean of a medical school (in which post optimism is essential for survival), I hope to approach in John Danz's spirit the five public health questions I have chosen to address.

Over the past forty years, so many people have contributed thoughts and ideas that have influenced me on the topics I have addressed that it would be impossible to acknowledge all of them. A partial listing of those to whom I am indebted would include Mort Lippmann, Mark Utell, Bernard Goldstein, Paul Lioy, Jack Spengler, Devra Davis, Scott Zeger, John Petkau, Geoffrey Rose, the late Donald Reid, the late Ronald Christie, Terry Anderson, Ronnie Sizto, Darrell Roberts, Bob Caton, Clyde Hertzmann, Peter Warren, Hans-Peter Witschi, David Rall, Arthur Upton, Larry Green, Fred Bass, Margaret Becklake, Charles Chapman, Bill McDonnell, Carl Hayes, David Mc-Kee, Les Grant, Andrew Churg, Corbett McDonald, Joel Schwartz, Bob Frank, Ben Ferris, Jim Whittenberger, Curtis Moore, Jim Pitts,

Tim Oke, Doug Dockery, Frank Speizer, Ira Tager, John Samet, Duncan Thomas, Sverre Vedal, Phil Landrigan, the late Irving Selikoff, Paul Brodeur, Fred Lipfert, Stephen Richman, Ed Wituschek, Jack Basuk, Ken Hare, Jim Ham, Gordon Butler, and Liora Salter.

I can recall stimulating discussions with members of the Epidemiology 2 study section of the National Institutes of Health, on which I served for four years; with members of the Science Council of Canada, of which I was a member for six years; with my fellow commissioners, Jim Murray, and the late Walter Raudsepp, on the Royal Commission on Uranium Mining in British Columbia; with Gene Matanoski, Pat Buffler, Donald Pierce, Barry Wilson, Kathleen Conway, Richard Wilson, Clark Heath, and other members of the committee convened by the Science Advisory Board of the U.S. Environmental Protection Agency to review data on electromagnetic fields; and with Don Hornig, John Bailar, Gil Omenn, and members of the Board of Environmental Studies of the National Academy of Sciences during my service on it.

I am also much indebted to the two reviewers to whom the University of Washington Press forwarded the first draft of the manuscript. Dr. Gil Omenn was one of these; the other was anonymous. Their questions and constructive suggestions led to important revisions in the text, with necessary expansion of some sections.

Needless to say, none of these individuals or organizations should accept any responsibility for the views I have expressed.

March 1993

Environmental Health Risks and Public Policy

1

Introduction

World War II was characterized by unparalleled suffering of the civilian population. Apart from the millions in military service who died in combat, millions of people were the targets of intensive air attacks in Rotterdam, London, Coventry, Dresden, Tokyo, and of course Hiroshima and Nagasaki; and millions of innocent civilians were summarily executed or gassed. After 1945, the world struggled back to normality from such cataclysmic events and the survivors turned themselves to the process of repair.

As a corporal in the Home Guard, I had been a witness in Kent of the Battle of Britain, and for most of the war was a medical student in or around London. I was in Hiroshima with the British army in March 1946. From 1948 to 1956 I was learning my specialty of lung physiology and lung disease, and, with others, I was looking after a special emphysema clinic at St. Bartholomew's Hospital in the center of the City of London. I date my interest in air pollution from the London episode of fog and severe air pollution in December 1952. This is the background to the chapters that follow. I was dissuaded from making them purely autobiographical by a note in a recent *New York Review of Books* that said, "Autobiography is, of course, the highest form of fiction."

It slowly became apparent after the war that there was much unfinished business that demanded attention. The four thousand excess deaths in London in December 1952 were a preliminary warning that air pollution could no longer be neglected. The public realized this earlier than the government of the day. The enormous acceleration in

3

the rate of cigarette smoking, which had occurred universally during the stress of the war, was not yet appreciated as the health disaster it would ultimately represent. Asbestos was recognized as a health risk to a few employees, and during the war the U.S. navy had issued some notes on the safe use of the material, but there is little evidence that any precautions were taken in its use (1). I saw my first case of fatal asbestosis from the Cape Asbestos plant in East Ham in 1949. Lead poisoning, occasionally seen in small children exposed to peeling, lead-containing paint, or in employees casting lead type for printing, was mentioned in medical school, but I do not recall seeing a recognized case of it. Any possible hazard of electromagnetic field exposure was not recognized.

The principal reason why exposures to these hazards have become a major focus of concern over the forty years since 1952 is that very large numbers of people have become exposed to some risk from them. Thus the catastrophic increase in cigarette smoking, which has only now begun to decline in some countries, led to an epidemic of lung cancer, emphysema, and heart disease. Air pollution, recognized as a possible problem locally when temperature inversions occurred, now affects very large numbers of people—in 1988, 86 million people in the United States were living in areas in which the ozone standard, based on health protection, was exceeded (2). The collapse of totalitarian regimes in eastern Europe revealed the presence of gross environmental degradation (3), much of it related to air pollution. At the present time in the Third World, acute respiratory disease is now the second commonest cause of death in children under five (4), and severe indoor and outdoor air contamination undoubtedly plays a major role in this (5).

In New York City, two-thirds of the 800,000 buildings apparently contain asbestos, and in many of these it is in poor condition (6). The widespread use of lead in gasoline everywhere (by 1967 the annual production of tetraethyl and tetramethyl lead in the United States for use in gasoline was 685 million pounds [7]) resulted in a fourfold increase in the lead content of snow strata samples in Greenland between 1940 and 1960 (see figure 2.10). The development of high voltage electrical transmission lines, together with the multiplicity of domestic appliances using electricity, must have greatly increased the general population's exposure to electromagnetic fields.

These observations indicate clearly that present concerns are not attributable to the energetic protestations of a lunatic environmental fringe, nor to the persistent obsession of the media with them. These concerns come about because of the very widespread dissemination of such hazards. We are generally aware of health risks because of the activities of the media, but it must be noted that media attention is episodic and much greater in relation to some of the hazards than to others. In addition, Rose has pointed out that a low level of exposure for a very large number of people may constitute a more serious public health problem than a higher level of exposure for a small group (8, 92), and this has to be kept constantly in mind.

In Chapter 2, I sketch each of these five hazards and the evolution of knowledge concerning them. These summaries are necessarily brief, but they are designed to illustrate the data that lie behind different judgments concerning each of them. I assess the role of the media, of scientists, of industry, of legislators, and of the courts in relation to each of the five, and some differences are noted between the free societies of Britain, Canada, and the United States in respect of them. Chapter 3 provides a detailed evaluation of five different problems that underlie contemporary policy decisions. Chapter 4 illustrates some common mistakes and misunderstandings, and examines the ways whereby a decision is made to protect the public health in a free society. In Chapter 5, I attempt to draw some conclusions as a guide to the future.

It is immediately apparent that such a review would require knowledge not only of lung disease, which I can claim to have, but also of child psychology (important in relation to the effects of lead), atmospheric chemistry, biostatistics, risk assessment, epidemiology, carcinogenesis, social sciences, political science, economics, and jurisprudence—fields in which I cannot claim expertise. However, it is my hope that I command a sufficient "defensive" knowledge of them that I can draw some useful general lessons.

2

Setting the Stage: Critical Risks

Table 2.1 lists sequentially the five hazards under discussion and compares them under twelve headings. This constitutes the underlying structure of the following discussion of each hazard.

It must be realized at the outset that each of these five topics is encompassed by an enormous bibliography. Many books have been devoted to each one separately. The summaries that follow are not designed to cover all the many aspects of the five hazards, but to bring out aspects of them that are important in any discussion of the public and legislative response that has been engendered.

Air Pollution

1952 was the year of the London smog episode, but concern about air pollution in that city stretched back almost four hundred years. It was often inferred, but not demonstrated, that air quality must be affecting health of the population, and there had been certain ominous signs. One of these was the occurrence in London in December of 1873 of an episode in which cattle died from the effects of a fog. This is described in a letter and an editorial in *The Veterinarian* in January 1874 (9). A Mr. Priestman noted that he was called to attend sick animals on the previous Tuesday and Wednesday during a heavy fog coincident with Cattle Show week in London. "On Tuesday, the first day of the fog, as early as eleven o'clock in the morning several animals were marked as affected with difficult breathing." By that evening "the majority of cattle in the Hall showed evidence of suffering. Sheep and pigs not affected. . . . On Wednesday, there was very little improve-ment in the atmospheric condition, and a large proportion of the cattle were so much distressed that it became necessary to do some-thing to satisfy the exhibitors, if not to relieve the animals." By Thurs-day things were better. Most of the animals were slaughtered, and "the post-mortem appearances were indicative of bronchitis; the mu-cous membrane of the smaller bronchial tubes was inflamed, and there was present the lobular congestion and emphysema which be-long to that disease." Many of the animals were noted to be febrile. *fever*

An editorial on page 32 of the same issue noted: "If any one, a few weeks ago, had suggested the possibility of a London fog doing seri-ous damage to cattle, or other animals, submitted to its influence, he would have been looked upon as supplying in himself a melancholy instance of intellectual fogginess." Such was the fate of Cassandra.

The great painter Claude Monet spent the winter of 1901 in Lon-don, and captured the foggy days in his paintings of Waterloo Bridge and Westminster. In an interview (10), he noted, "The fog in London assumes all sorts of colours; there are black, brown, yellow, green, purple fogs, and the interest in painting is to get the objects as seen through all these fogs. My practised eye has found that objects change in appearance in a London fog more and quicker than in any other atmosphere, and the difficulty is to get every change down on canvas." Another commentator (10) quoted him as remarking that London was much more beautiful than the English countryside, but only in winter, when the fogs gave it a magnificent sense of space by obscuring detail. He painted more than a hundred canvases of Water-loo Bridge, Charing Cross Bridge, and the Houses of Parliament; it has been noted that (10) "the paintings show the foggy river and city surrounding it under gray skies or when the sun penetrated the fog or illuminated smoke." Contemporary coal-burning air pollution played a major part in producing these effects, which Monet so successfully caught in his paintings.

The 1952 episode in London occurred between December 5 and 8. As the later official government report on the episode (11) noted, "The fog was notable for its density and its duration and an important feature was the almost complete absence of remissions, either in den-sity or in temperature, during the four days. In a city traditionally notorious for its fogs, there was general agreement on its exceptional severity on this occasion." An appendix to that report noted that the

Table 2.1. Summary of Five Environmental Hazards

	Air Pollution	Cigarettes	Asbestos	Lead	Electromagnetic Fields
Year*	1952	1963	1975	1980	1986
Significant Outcomes	Episodes: long-term effects	Lung cancer; COPD heart disease	Mesothelioma; lung cancer (asbestosis)	Children: cognitive defect; adults: hypertension	Children: leukemia; adults: cancers
Strength of Epidemiol Data	Indirect indices; variable associations	Very strong	Very strong	Difficult outcome to evaluate; moderately strong	Associations: difficult to assess causal relationship
Low Exposures	Chronic effects	Environmental tobacco smoke	As in buildings; risk is controversial	?Effects with blood levels 15–30 dL/L	No dose response data
Exposure Measurement	Not precise	Fair in smokers; passive dose difficult	Very difficult in most cases	Deduced from biomarkers	Very difficult; deduced from surrogates such as wiring configuration

Role of Acute Episodes	+	Nil	Nil	Nil	Nil
Type of Risk	Involuntary	Voluntary/involuntary	Involuntary	Involuntary	Involuntary
Public Perception of Risk vs. Numerical Estimate	?	Low	High	Low	?High
Industry Involved	Automobile; electric power	Tobacco; advertising	Mining; insulation secondary industry	Petrochemical; automobile	Electric utilities
Media Coverage	Intermittent (strong in Los Angeles)	Intermittent	Intermittent	Not extensive	Recently strong
Legislative Response	Yes	Yes	Yes	Yes	Not yet
Involvement of Courts/Lawyers	Absent	Not major	Dominant	Absent; ?starting	Increasing

*Approximate year of first major public concern.

Smithfield Club's show was being held at Earl's Court in London over those days, and sixty cattle needed veterinary attention on account of respiratory symptoms, with one dying and twelve having to be slaughtered. The writers of the report referred to the similar episode in 1873. The report noted the episodes of air pollution from industrial sources with human mortality in the Meuse Valley in 1931, and in Donora in Pennsylvania in 1948.

In the case of the London episode, it was realized within a few days that there had been a major increase in daily mortality. In the House of Commons, a written question was tabled soon after the episode, and a written reply was given on 18 December 1952. In this, the Health Minister, Iain MacLeod, stated that the deaths in greater London during the week ending December 13 were 4, 703, compared with 1,852 in the corresponding week of 1951. Hospital admissions for the week ending on December 12 were 2,007 compared with 917 in the comparable week in 1951. He stated, "The cold weather had already caused some increase, but a large part of these increases must be attributed to the fog." On the same day, a question was asked, "Is there enough evidence to justify more energetic research into the harmful constituents of the air in towns?" The mortality and air pollution data in the episode are shown in figure 2.1.

By 23 January 1953, more persistent questions were being asked. Harold MacMillan, then the Minister of Housing and Local Government, parried these, but his attitude must have seemed too little concerned, since a member asked, "Does the Minister not appreciate that last month, in Greater London alone, there were literally more people choked to death by air pollution than were killed on the roads in the whole country in 1952? Why is a public inquiry not being held?" Mr. MacMillan stated: "I am not satisfied that further general legislation is needed at present. I am however keeping this aspect of the matter in hand."

The newspapers continued their criticism of government inaction. I can recall a meeting occurring at this time between Professor Ronald Christie, who headed the Professorial Medical Unit at St. Bartholomew's Hospital, and a couple of senior civil servants from the Ministry of Health. They were trying to draft a reassuring response to be given in the House of Commons to a question on action following the episode. One of the civil servants read out a sentence he had been drafting that said something about a "new research initiative," which

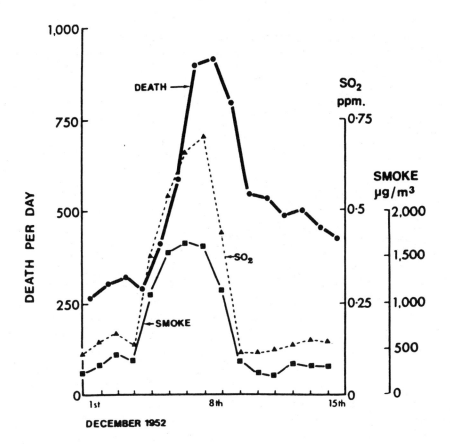

Figure 2.1. Air pollution levels and excess mortality in London in December 1952. The smoke level of more than 1500 micrograms/m^3 reduced visibility to a few yards. One SO$_2$ monitor recorded levels of more than 1.00 part per million (ppm) at the height of the episode. The daily death rate did not return to its normal level of about 270 deaths per day for a further two weeks. Redrawn from reference 14.

had been taken "at one of London's oldest hospitals." Ronald Christie said, "That's a bonnie phrase and has the added advantage of being true." His candor scandalized the bureaucrats.

Rereading the exchanges in the House of Commons, one is impressed by the general lack of discussion as to which constituents of the fog might have been harmful, and where they came from. As a result of a continuing sense of public outrage at the inaction of the government (as expressed by the newspapers), the government finally established the Beaver Committee in July 1953; and it was this committee's report that led to the clean air legislation in 1956. Lord Ashby, reviewing these events (12), noted the initial apathy of the government, and made the important comment that the Beaver Committee succeeded in proposing successful legislation that enabled local authorities to forbid open coal burning because alternative smokeless fuels were available for immediate use.

In the United States, a similar growth in public awareness of air pollution's health effects began to lead to legislation to curb its worst constituents. Professor Joel Tarr (13), of the Carnegie-Mellon Institute, has documented in detail the steps taken in Pittsburgh that led to passage in 1946 of a city ordinance against air pollution. A group of citizens, including a physician, started a campaign in 1941 for clean air legislation. Making little headway by public argument, they decided that the city council would have to be replaced; by 1946 they had succeeded both in doing this and in passing an air pollution ordinance. They relied on stories about the adverse impacts on public health in their campaign, but no scientific evidence was available that these were actually occurring. Dr. Hope Alexander, the physician member of the citizen group, was Director of the Pittsburgh Department of Health. He was quoted as saying, in 1941, "The medical profession is in accord with the statement that smoke is a health menace of major proportions. . . . For the present, however, there are few scientific facts to definitely establish a case of cause and effect." Various groups, including the League of Women Voters and several women's clubs, the board of trade of a wealthy Pittsburgh neighborhood, and the members of the activist group, all took a prominent role in getting the ordinance passed. This was an era in which simple assertion was all that was expected—that is, before epidemiological data were required as a basis for such opinions.

In 1970, a report for the Royal College of Physicians of London on air pollution and health appeared (14), and in the same year, after a long period of U.S. Senate hearings and discussion, the first clean air act was passed in the United States. Human health concerns played a prominent part in motivating legislators to control air pollution at this time.

The sequence—of effective legislation resulting from a single disaster and public pressure on a government to deal with it—appears to be the exception rather than the rule. As will be noted later, it is much more difficult to get legislative action against lower level but repetitive exposure to air pollutants. Nevertheless, by 1970, plenty of evidence indicated that uncontrolled coal burning, with high particulate and SO_2 emissions, was damaging.

In the same year as the London episode, a chemist in Los Angeles worked out for the first time the chemical reactions that led to the formation of ozone from oxides of nitrogen in the presence of hydrocarbons and sunlight—the generation of so-called "photochemical smog" (15). In the 1960s, work began to establish the acute effects of ozone on people and on plants and crops. In modern cities, most of the oxide of nitrogen from which ozone is formed is emitted by automobiles. Initially, this problem was thought to be confined to Los Angeles, because that is where most of the monitoring of the air for photochemical oxidant pollution was being routinely carried out. It is now recognized to be a serious problem over most of Europe, in North America, and even in Australia.

Contemporary perceptions of air pollution can be summarized as follows:

1. In eastern Europe and in much of the Third World, particularly in China, gross particulate and sulphur dioxide pollution is occurring. This is believed to have long-term adverse effects on both children and adults. The first satisfactory epidemiological study of the effects of living in this kind of pollution was published in London in 1965 (16). It took account of cigarette smoking, and, by studying employees of the British Post Office, standardized the socioeconomic level of the population being studied. It found convincing evidence that lung function was lower in men who lived in greater London than in men who lived in smaller country towns, where sulfur dioxide levels and particulate pollution were less than half what they were in London. This kind of pollution leads to higher levels of chronic bronchitis and possibly also of asthma. The effect of living in the pollution is interactive with cigarette smoking. The basic data from this study are shown in figure 2.2. Very similar data—as a consequence of air pollution from open coal combustion—are now being reported from China (17). The forced expiratory volume in liters (FEVl), a simple test of lung function, was shown to be significantly lower in nonsmoking women in Beijing if they lived in zones of the city with higher particulate and SO_2 pollution. A lower FEVl in such cross-sectional studies in those living in more polluted regions might be caused by a faster rate of

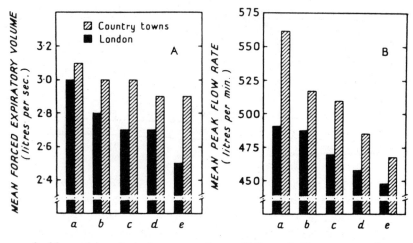

—A, **Mean forced expiratory volume (1·0 sec.); B, mean peak flow-rate (both standardised to age 40).**

(*a*) non-smokers, (*b*) ex-smokers, (*c*) smokers, 1–14 g. per day, (*d*) smokers, 15–24 g. per day, (*e*) smokers, 25 g. or more per day.

Mean value and number of subjects:

A, (*a*) 3·1 (30) & 3·0 (13); (*b*) 3·0 (77) & 2·8 (36); (*c*) 3·0 (142) & 2·7 (74); (*d*) 2·9 (134) & 2·7 (98); (*e*) 2·9 (40) & 2·5 (29).

B, (*a*) 562 (31) & 491 (13); (*b*) 517 (77) & 488 (36); (*c*) 510 (142) & 470 (74); (*d*) 485 (134) & 458 (98); (*e*) 468 (41) & 448 (29).

Figure 2.2. Cross-sectional study of lung function in British postal workers in 1965. From reference 16. At that time SO_2 and smoke levels in the country towns were about half those in London. Note that the largest differences in forced expiratory volume in liters (FEV1) between the London and country dwellers were in the heaviest smoking category. The peak flow rates are very different in the nonsmoking category, but the numbers are small.

decline of lung function with age, or the presence of subclinical lung changes changes, or the fact that children living in polluted air never attain the same "normal" value for this test in early adult life; or, of course, to all three of these effects.

2. Photochemical air pollution is now known to be much commoner than previously realized. The U.S. Clean Air Act of 1970 required the development of standards for the protection of public health. In the case of ozone, this standard was initially set at 0.08 ppm for one hour, but later was revised upwards to its present level of 0.12 ppm. The Canadian standard remained at 0.08 ppm. In 1988, 86 mil-

lion Americans were living in areas where the 0.12 ppm standard was transgressed (2). Ozone is an intensely irritant gas, and lung function is adversely affected in young normal subjects if they exercise in 0.08 ppm for six hours (18). Ozone acts by inducing inflammation in the lung (19, 20). It is considered to be a special hazard to asthmatics, because the effect on lung function and on airway responsiveness is exerted on lungs that are already abnormal in these aspects (21). Photochemical pollution is a major problem in many Third World countries, and some of the highest levels now occurring are in Mexico City. We still know very little about long-term adverse effects on people of living in an oxidant environment. Crop yields, of such things as alfalfa grass and beans, are depressed by ozone exposure below the current standards during the growing season.

3. When sulfur dioxide emissions occur in the presence of ozone formation, sulphuric acid aerosol is formed and can be directly detected in the air (18). This is later neutralized by ammonia to form sulphates. It is these aerosols that limit summer visibility over much of the northeastern North American continent. This summer acid haze, with ozone and ammonium sulphate, has been shown to be associated with increased hospital admissions for acute respiratory disease (23). These data are shown in figure 2.3 and in table 2.2. New data from the summers of 1986, 1987, and 1988 from Toronto have confirmed these findings (25).

4. Automobiles, trucks, and buses emit oxides of nitrogen and fine particulates. These are less than 10 microns in size and of complex composition. Under inversion conditions, they remain suspended in the air, and form a visible blanket enveloping a city and obliterating adjacent mountains. Recent studies have indicated that increases in this form of pollution are regularly associated with increases in total mortality; this has now been shown to be true of eleven different locations with widely differing climatic conditions (26). Recent data for Philadelphia are shown in table 2.3 and in figures 2.4 and 2.5. The mechanism of this effect is currently unknown. It may be observed that reducing general automobile pollution is a much more complex problem than the reduction of particulate pollution from coal burning required in 1953.

5. Most discussions of the effects of air pollution on health are centered on the interpretation of epidemiological data. Studies of controlled acute human exposures have proved very important in defining

Table 2.2. Pearson Correlation Coefficients for July and August Admissions in Southern Ontario for Years 1974 and 1976–1983 Based on Deviations from Same Day of Week in Same Season in Same Year

			Diagnostic Category			
Variable	Total	Respiratory	Respiratory Minus Asthma	Asthma All ages	Asthma 0–14	Non-respiratory
SO$_2$ L0	ns[a]	ns	ns	ns	ns	ns
SO$_2$ L24	ns	ns	ns	ns	ns	ns
SO$_2$ L48	ns	0.1383**	0.1125*	0.1063*	ns	ns
O$_3$ L0	0.1217*	ns	ns	ns	ns	ns
O$_3$ L24	ns	0.1374**	ns	0.1241*	ns	ns
O$_3$ L48	ns	0.1469**	0.1492*	ns	ns	ns
NO$_2$ L0	0.1137*	ns	ns	ns	ns	ns
NO$_2$ L24	ns	ns	ns	ns	ns	ns
NO$_2$ L48	ns	0.1102*	ns	ns	ns	ns
COH L0	0.1586**	ns	ns	ns	ns	ns
COH L24	ns	ns	ns	ns	ns	ns
COH L48	ns	ns	ns	ns	ns	ns
SO$_4$ L0	ns	ns	ns	ns	ns	ns
SO$_4$ L24	ns	0.1706**	0.1341*	0.1265*	ns	ns
SO$_4$ L48	ns	0.1339*	0.1290*	ns	ns	ns
T L0	0.1081*	ns	0.1069*	ns	ns	ns
T L24	ns	ns	0.1344**	ns	ns	ns
T L48	ns	0.1286*	0.1681**	ns	ns	ns
RH L0	ns	ns	ns	ns	ns	ns
RH L24	ns	ns	ns	ns	ns	ns
RH L48	ns	ns	ns	ns	ns	ns

[a]ns = Not significant.

* $P \leq 0.01$.

**$P \leq 0.001$.

From reference 23. The simplest way of showing nonrandom associations between two variables, in this case hospital respiratory admissions (as a percentage deviation from the mean value for that day of the week in the same season of the same year), and for the mean of the hourly maxima for the pollutant for all monitors in the region. The associations are significant in spite of the maximally conservative data selection (since the mean value to which each day is compared is affected by any pollution-related admissions).

a minimum-effects level of single gaseous pollutants, and in establishing that some individuals are much more sensitive than others to certain pollutants (asthmatics being an order of magnitude more sensitive to the acute effects of sulfur dioxide than are nonasthmatics, for example). Animal exposure studies throw light on biological plausibility and mechanisms of action. They are also the only way in which possible long-term effects can be experimentally studied.

    6. It has been difficult to establish with any certainty the long-term adverse effects of living in a polluted atmosphere. The cross-sectional

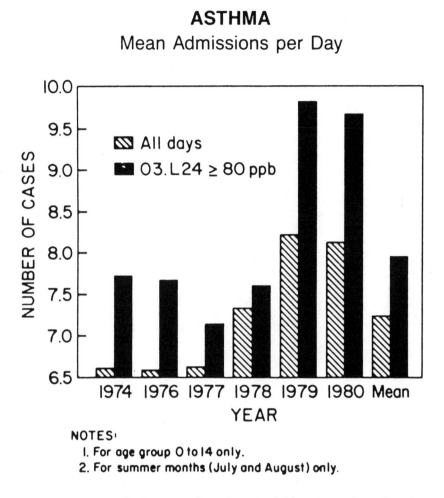

ASTHMA
Mean Admissions per Day

NOTES:
1. For age group 0 to 14 only.
2. For summer months (July and August) only.

Figure 2.3. Hospital admissions for asthma in children in southern Ontario, 1974–1980. From reference 24. From the same data as in table 2.2. These data for asthma admissions in children aged 0–14 show a consistent excess in mean admissions 24 hours after the ozone level (as a mean of the hourly maxima) exceeded the Canadian standard of 80 parts per billion.

study by Holland and Reid in Britain in 1965 (16) showed that lung function was lower in men in a more polluted region (see figure 2.2); this constitutes one of the more convincing pieces of evidence of long-term effects in the general population. It is possible that the observation is to be explained by the adverse effects of pollutants on children,

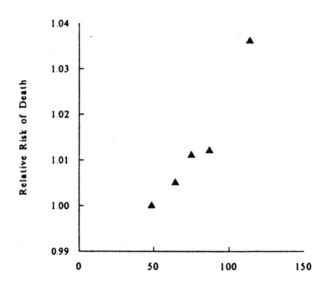

Total Suspended Particulates

Relative risk of death in Philadelphia by quintile
of total suspended particulates controlling by regression for year of study, time trend, and weather.

Figure 2.4. Relative risk of death in Philadelphia in relation to particulates. From the same data as table 2.3 (reference 26). Note than an increase from about 50 to 120 micrograms/m^3 in pollution is associated with about a 4 percent increase in mortality.

so that in polluted areas the population never reaches the same level of "normality" of pulmonary function as do children growing up in a clean environment. Such effects as shortened survival provide very crude indices of effects; and major disbenefits must have occurred before such an index would change significantly. Differences in respiratory disease incidence or in mortality in cross-sectional comparisons are difficult to interpret unless cigarette smoking is precisely known, since this is such a dominant factor in the causation of chronic respiratory disease. Even passive smoke inhalation has to be considered in this context.

This very brief summary of current knowledge leads to the following conclusions:

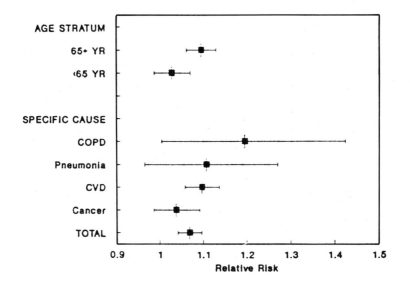

Figure 2.5. Relative risk of mortality in Philadelphia associated with a 100 microgram/m^3 increase in total suspended particulates (TSP) concentration after controlling by regression for year of study, time trend, and weather. Results for all-cause mortality, age-stratified mortality, and cause-specific mortality. From the same database as table 2.3 and figure 2.4 (reference 26). Note the increased risk of death from chronic obstructive pulmonary disease and pneumonia; however, together these account for only about one-tenth as many deaths as cardiovascular disease (see table 2.3). Numerically, the 10 percent increase in relative risk for cardiovascular disease when there is a 100 microgram/m^3 increase in particulate pollution is more important in driving the overall relationship.

1. Intense media attention can be generated by a single major episode of air pollution, but it is much harder to get the attention of legislators in order to deal with long-term, unspectacular, chronic effects. Yet, in the long run, these may be the more important.

2. As noted in table 2.1, in almost all studies of air pollution effects the actual exposure of the subject is very poorly characterized. To some extent this is inevitable if a large population is involved.

3. Air pollution generally represents an involuntary risk. Some avoidance may be possible by staying indoors. Some segments of the population, such as children returning from school at a time when ozone concentrations are highest, or young adults taking vigorous

Table 2.3. Daily Mortality Counts, Weather, and Air Pollution in Philadelphia, 1973–1980

	5%	10%	25%	50%	75%	90%	95%	Mean
Weather								
Temperature, °F	25	30	41	56	71	77	80	54.8
Dew Point, °F	9	15	28	44	59	68	70	42.8
Air pollutants								
TSP, $\mu g/m^3$	37	43	56	73	94	117	132	77.2
SO_2, ppb	6	8	12	18	27	39	46	21.0
Mortality, deaths/ day								
Total	35	37	42	48	54	60	64	48.2
Age ≤ 65 yr	10	11	14	17	20	23	25	16.9
Age > 65 yr	21	23	26	31	36	40	44	31.3
Cause-specific mortality, deaths/day								
Cardiovascular	13	15	18	22	26	30	32	22.1
Cancer	5	6	8	10	13	15	16	10.5
Pneumonia	0	0	0	1	2	3	4	1.44
Chronic obstructive pulmonary disease	0	0	0	1	1	2	3	0.89

exercise in polluted atmospheres, must be presumed to get much higher exposures than others.

4. It is not possible to estimate whether the public perception of the current risks posed by air pollution is generally higher or lower than statistical estimates. In any community with any air pollution problem, there is a cadre of interested citizens prepared to urge the importance of its amelioration. There are special problems in the Third World. A recent World Bank report (22) noted, "The potential constituency in favor of air pollution control is weakly identifiable and poorly informed of the causes, possible effects, and available technological alternatives. In contrast, those against pollution control enforcement are economically powerful and politically well organized."

5. Major industries interested in air pollution legislation are coal-burning electric utilities, the mining industry that produces the coal, and the automobile industry and the fuel suppliers for automobile transport. These have generally mounted strong opposition to more stringent controls or to tighter standards. The American Petroleum Institute in the United States a few years ago apparently spent several million dollars to oppose the proposed ozone standard.

6. Media coverage tends to be intermittent. In Los Angeles, a complex system of public alerts in relation to the level of oxidant pollution

makes the public aware of the pollution situation on a day-to-day basis. Similar daily reports on air quality now exist in many cities. A recent (December 14 and 15, 1991) oxide of nitrogen pollution episode in London led to public warnings carried in newspapers and on the radio. In North America, readings of various "air pollution indices" are routinely published and publicized.

7. In western Europe and North America, clean air legislation introduced between 1956 and 1970 has led to a major diminution in SO_2 and gross particulate pollution. Although in 1960 pollutant emission levels were not much different between western and eastern Europe, by 1990 many regions in eastern Europe were grossly polluted, whereas in western Europe these forms of pollution had been greatly reduced and were under control. The latest U.S. Clean Air Act amendments (1990) are expected to reduce sulfur dioxide emissions still further. In most democratic societies, there has been a legislative response to the public demand for clean air.

8. The American Lung Association has led public pressure for effective legislation to control air pollution in the United States. In Canada, a special coalition was formed to fight acid rain. The strong public support for this exerted some pressure on the Canadian government to try to persuade the U.S. government of the need for joint legislative action.

9. As noted in table 2.1, in general, courts and lawyers have not been much involved in the process of air pollution control. However, they have been extensively involved in hazardous-waste site litigation, and in some cases of localized release of toxic air pollutants. In Japan, unique legislation permitted legal suits between victims of air pollution (who not surprisingly proved to be very numerous) and primary emitters.

Environmental groups, together with the American Lung Association, have recently filed a suit against the U.S. Environmental Protection Agency (EPA) complaining that the agency has not moved to consider revision of the ozone standard in the light of new scientific information (some of it originating in the laboratories of the EPA itself). It is possible that, in the future, the courts may be more involved in such questions in the United States, but in a parliamentary system, as noted below, there would be no grounds for any such action.

We may fairly conclude that public opinion has been important in the control of air pollution; that it is difficult to deal with noncatastrophic events; that current air pollution is much more complex in origin and effects than was formerly the case; that biological plausibility varies with different combinations of pollutants; that there has been relatively little involvement of the legal process, and media interest is generally local; and that there are significant present and future problems in the Third World in relation to indoor and outdoor air pollution.

Cigarette Smoking

In table 2.1, I have dated concern about cigarette smoking to the date of publication of the first U.S. Surgeon General's report on the effects of smoking, which appeared in 1964. A report of the Royal College of Physicians of London had appeared two years earlier documenting the adverse effects of smoking. The history of cigarette smoking is as replete with statistical information as is baseball. In the following summary, some of the salient landmarks are identified.

The sociological history of cigarette smoking has many interesting facets. In about 1880, the popular Victorian painter T. J. Frith painted a large canvas of a young man lighting a cigarette for a rather gaudily attired young lady. Probably painted in the Tivoli Gardens in Copenhagen, the picture was entitled *Her First Cigarette*. It was one of a series of paintings with moral messages, but was deemed too obscene for public display. At about the same time, Van Gogh painted a remarkable canvas of a skeleton with a cigarette between its jaws. This picture is very rarely reproduced; perhaps the tobacco companies managed to get it suppressed.

The design of automated machinery for cigarette manufacture was perfected in 1913; the American Cancer Society was founded in the same year (28). A Canadian text on human physiology for use in schools, published in 1930 (29), contained dire warnings of the evil consequences of smoking. It stated that smoking leads to moral degeneration, and asserted (without giving a reference) that the reformatories and prisons were full of cigarette smokers. Unfortunately, the dangers of lung disease were not mentioned.

Cigarette consumption rose steadily but slowly until World War II, when in all countries there was a major acceleration of the rate of smoking. Epidemiological studies, including a prospective study of British doctors, began in about 1950. The first disease to be linked unequivocally to cigarette consumption was lung cancer. The causal significance of the association was immediately challenged. Sir Ronald Fisher, a leading British biostatistician, a Fellow of the prestigious Royal Society, and a pioneer in the statistics of experimental design, was prominent in suggesting that there was no causal link between cigarettes and lung cancer. Only recently has it become known that he was being paid for his activities by the tobacco industry (30).

By the time of the publication of the U.S. Surgeon General's report in 1964, there was overwhelming evidence that cigarette smoking was strongly associated with lung cancer, chronic obstructive lung disease, peripheral vascular disease, and heart disease. The causal relationship was no longer doubted by the majority of physicians, and further epidemiological studies were hardly required.

Recent data indicate that adverse effects are even associated with passive inhalation of cigarette smoke (33). In 1986, both the National Academy of Sciences (31) and the U.S. Department of Health and Human Services (32) issued summary reports on the effects of passive tobacco smoke inhalation. I was at a meeting in Germany in 1988 at which there was a session on passive tobacco effects (33). (A distinguished, but very elderly, American biostatistician was flown over to tell us that the evidence of causality in such studies was too flimsy to be believed.) The observation that passive smoke inhalation was capable of causing ill effects had the effect of changing completely the basis for legislation, since cigarette smoke was no longer only a voluntary risk. Prohibition of smoking in commercial aircraft, workplaces, and restaurants quickly followed.

In Britain, cigarette consumption reached a peak in the mid-1960s; thereafter it fell in men but continued to rise in women (34). In the United States, smoking peaked in 1963, when per capita consumption in persons over the age of 18 reached 4250 cigarettes per year (35). In the United States in 1965, 13 percent of women smoked more than 25 cigarettes a day; by 1985 this had risen to 23 percent (36). The reasons for this increase are largely unknown, but may well be attributable to a clever advertising campaign aimed at the self-image of young women.

The disease burden attributable to cigarette consumption is enormous. It has been calculated that a 25 year old smoking two packs/day loses 8.3 years of expected longevity; this works out to five and a half minutes of life lost per cigarette smoked (37). Direct adverse health costs of smoking in the United States have been estimated at $16 billion a year, with indirect costs more than double that figure (37). The disease burden attributable to smoking far outweighs the combined effects of the other hazards I have chosen to consider. Sir Richard Doll (38), writing in 1983, concluded:

> The avoidance of smoking would alone reduce the mortality from all cancers by about a third (including avoidance of not only the large majority of cancers of the mouth, throat, and lung, but also a substantial proportion of the deaths attributed to cancers of the bladder, kidney, and pancreas). It would almost eliminate chronic obstructive lung disease and the complications of peripheral vascular disease, would reduce the age specific mortality from aortic aneurysm by at least three quarters and the mortality from myocardial infarction by about a quarter, and would probably lead to a small reduction in perinatal mortality in the poorer socioeconomic groups.

Furthermore, concomitant cigarette smoking greatly increases the risk of lung cancer in asbestos- or radon-exposed workers. This question is discussed in more detail in Chapter 3.

Since 1964, in many countries public societies have been established to reinforce government campaigns against the tobacco industry. There is convincing evidence that measures taken—including prevention of television advertising and progressively more severe taxation—have had an effect. It is now calculated, for example, that whereas in 1989 annual adult per capita cigarette consumption in the United States would have been fifty-five hundred cigarettes without preventive measures, the actual figure was about three thousand (39). The percentage of men who smoked reached a high of 69 percent in 1958, but by 1989 this was down to 30 percent (39). In Britain, lung cancer rates in men have peaked and have begun to decline, but they are still rising in young women. However, the lung cancer rates in women of all ages began to fall in about 1970 (see figure 2.6) (34). The same is broadly true for chronic obstructive lung disease mortality.

The diminution of cigarette consumption in free societies has not been uniform. Reasons for the differences between these countries are obscure, but they may be a reflection of different media emphasis.

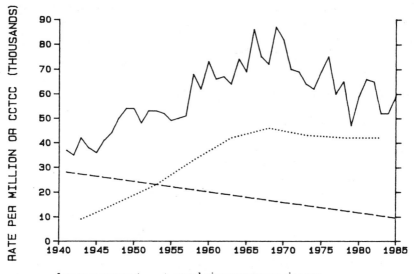

Lung cancer rate (——), cumulative constant tar cigarette consumption (CCTCC .....), and hypothesised "background" rate of lung cancer unrelated to cigarette consumption (— — —), for women aged 40–44, 1941–85.

Figure 2.6. Changing patterns of lung cancer mortality and cigarette smoking in women in Britain. From reference 34. Although air pollution began to decline in the UK from about 1965 onwards, the authors do not consider that the decline in lung cancer might be due to this factor, but instead that the rise in lung cancer in women from 1940 to 1970 occurred against a falling background rate of lung cancer unrelated to cigarettes.

Table 2.4 shows the changes in smoking rates in different countries between 1974 and 1987 (40). It has been difficult in democratic societies to define what steps can be taken against a product that can legally be sold. Lawsuits brought by the relatives of victims of lung cancer against the tobacco industry have generally not succeeded. In Canada, a recent court decision upheld the right of the government to restrict tobacco advertising, and there are current proposals to require licensing of sellers of tobacco and to outlaw cigarette machines from public places. Campaigns in high schools about the dangers of cigarette smoking may have had some effect, but the increasing rate of smoking among young women has not been halted. Perhaps there was more sense to the banning of the display of Frith's painting than one might have thought.

Table 2.4. International Comparisons of Trends in Cigarette
Smoking Prevalence

MEN aged 20 and over: % smoking						
YEAR	USA	GB	Australia	Canada	Norway	Sweden
1974–6	43.4	52	43.3	45.6	49.6	36
1983	35.5	38	38.9	35.7	44.6	26
1986–7	31.7	35	32.9	32.3	41.3	24
WOMEN aged 20 and over: %smoking						
YEAR	USA	GB	Australia	Canada	Norway	Sweden
1974–5	31.4	41	31.9	32	32.1	34
1982–3	29.4	34	31.4	29.3	32.3	28
1986–7	26.8	31	30.6	26.6	33.3	27

In every country, the higher the education level, the lower the smoking prevalence.

From reference 40. Note the higher declines in women in smoking in the United Kingdom, Canada, and the United States, compared to Australia and Norway. This might be due to differences in media impact.

Media emphasis on the health effects of cigarette smoking has been variable. Initially, the press generally underemphasized the risk, fearing loss of advertising revenue. The tobacco industry, with enormous profits, commands such a powerful potential (used historically to "buy" some scientific testimony or to pay for influential back-room lobbying in political circles) that it is not easy to combat it. The income from tobacco taxation is important for many governments, further inhibiting effective legislation. In many countries, tobacco advertising still succeeds in getting a message across to the insecure teenager that smoking is an important symbol of adult independence.

Cigarette advertising and promotion in the Third World is generally unrestricted, and, as consumption has declined in the industrialized countries, tobacco consumption has been aggressively promoted by the tobacco industry in lesser developed nations. In China, the late Chairman Mao was rarely photographed without a cigarette in his hand, so public health emphasis on the dangers of smoking was impossible. More recently in China, some public education on the dangers of smoking has been initiated.

In the case of cigarette smoking, the epidemiological data are now more or less complete; initially, the causative inference was contested; there have been significant government initiatives in most western countries; the issues now are psychosocial and legal, and in all jurisdictions problems exist in limiting advertising and promotion; and currently there is an intensive push by tobacco companies to increase sales in the developing world. Pierce (41) has recently noted that the overseas sales of American cigarettes doubled between 1986 and 1989. He attributes this, at least in part, to the fact that cigarette manufacture "is increasingly becoming an oligopoly controlled by four large transnational companies and the government of China."

Asbestos

A great deal has been written about the remarkable history of asbestos. Commercial production started in about 1880, and by 1920 world production was about two hundred thousand tons annually. By 1940 this had about doubled; but a step increase to about a million tons a year occurred during World War II. Part of this was accounted for by the extensive use of asbestos in ships. However, general use had also been rising steadily: the United States–manufactured steam locomotive of the 1930s contained three thousand pounds of asbestos (42). After 1950, production growth rose continuously till 1970, when it amounted to about 4 million tons per year. In the building boom of the 1950s, asbestos was widely applied within buildings as a sprayed fire retardant. The growth in the number of automobiles, for which asbestos was required for brake linings, was also part of this expansion. As noted in the introduction, currently two-thirds of the eight hundred thousand buildings in Manhattan are believed to contain asbestos, and in many the mineral is in poor condition, being friable and easily dispersed (6).

Becklake (43) has plotted this growth of asbestos production with the evolution of medical knowledge in relation to its effects (see figure 2.7). That it was capable of causing irreversible lung changes was already known in the 1930s. Its relationship to lung cancer was clearly established only forty years later, and it was not until the mid-1960s that the entity of pleural mesothelioma was defined. The major conference convened by the International Agency for Research in Cancer (IARC) in 1972 (44) provides a useful milestone in the evolution of modern knowledge. By that time, the increased incidence of mesothelioma in port cities around the world as a result of ship repair work was well established. It also became clear that a mesothelioma could result from relatively high exposure over a short period of time. From this date, the relative dangers of the different forms of asbestos became a major question, not wholly resolved even today.

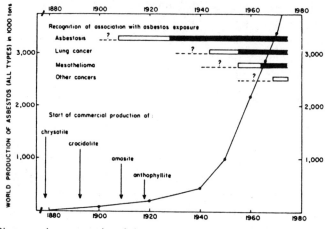

Diagrammatic representation of the growth of the asbestos industry and the recognition of the associated biologic effects. The following symbols indicate the association with asbestos: ? = suspected; ☐ = probable; ■ = established.

Figure 2.7. Asbestos production and the evolution of medical knowledge. From reference 43. Since 1980, there has been a considerable reduction in world use of asbestos, but, as noted in the text, mesothelioma incidence in some countries is still rising.

The forced bankruptcy in 1982 of the United States' major producer of asbestos—as a result of the many outstanding injury claims that had been filed against it—has been documented in detail by Paul Brodeur (45). The role of the asbestos industry and of the lawyers representing it, in fighting allegations of responsibility, constituted a remarkable indictment (not contested in any lawsuit against the author of the book).

As indicated in table 2.1, the epidemiological data in relation to asbestos are very strong and come from many countries. The progressive decline in maximal exposure standards for asbestos fibers from 1946 to 1990, as shown in table 2.5, indicates the progressive awareness of the risks from inhaling the material. As shown, in 1968 the American Council of Governmental and Industrial Hygienists (ACGIH) standard was 12 fibers per milliliter (ml) of air; and in 1990 the U.S. Occupational Safety and Health Administration (OSHA) standard was 0.1 fibers/ml, a drop of more than a hundred-fold (4). The precise risk attendant on use of buildings that contain asbestos is still controversial, and measure-

Table 2.5. Recommended Air Concentration Limits and Standards for Asbestos

Group	Year	Limit
ACGIH	1946	5×10^6 particles/ft^3
ACGIHG	1968[a]	12 fibers[c]/mL or 2×10^6 particles/ft^3
ACGIH	1970,[a] 1974[b]	5 fibers/mL
OSHA	1972	5 fibers/mL
OSHA	1976	2 fibers/mL
NIOSH	1976	0.1 fiber/mL
ACGIH	1978,[a] 1980[b]	0.2 fiber/mL for crocidolite
		0.5 fiber/mL for amosite
		2.0 fiber/mL for chrysotile and other forms
OSHA	1976	2.0 fiber/mL
	1986	0.2 fiber/mL
	1990 proposal	0.1 fiber/mL

[a]Notice of intent.

[b]Adopted as threshold limit value (TLV).

[c]All fiber limits based on phase-contrast optical determination at 400–450× magnification.

From reference 46. Over this period, standards for many other hazardous materials, such as lead and benzene, have also fallen.

ment of exposure in this situation is very difficult (see table 2.6). The risk is usually involuntary.

Although to my knowledge it has not been quantified, the public perception of the risk from asbestos may be higher than the published numerical estimates. Both primary producers and secondary industries have been implicated in perceived risk. Media coverage has been very intermittent; some vivid descriptive television documentaries were prepared in the early 1980s, but the subject is now rarely mentioned in the media except in relation to local issues (usually related to contentious litigation). There has, however, been considerable discussion in the media in relation to local issues, for example the pressure on local school boards to insist on the removal of all asbestos from schools regardless of its physical state or the dangers it represents.

What distinguishes the present status of asbestos as a health hazard in the United States is the dominant role played by the courts and the legal profession. The financial outcomes are so large and the cost of asbestos removal (if done safely) is so considerable that many major lawsuits have taken place or are in process. These have required

Table 2.6. Distribution of Building Average Airborne Asbestos Concentrations for Nonlitigation Data by Study[a]

Study	No. of Buildings	Building Types[b]	Minimum	10th Percentile	Median	Mean	90th Percentile	Maximum
Burdett and Jaffrey 1986[c]	39	5S,8PC,26R	0	0	0.0001	0.00026	0.0009	0.0017
Chatfield 1986	7	5S,2PC	0	0	0.0005	0.00243	0.0080	0.0080
Gazzi and Crockford 1987[c]	25	R	0	0	0	0.00030	0.0008	0.0025
Hatfield et al. 1988; Chesson et al. 1990b; Crump and Farrar 1989	43	PC	0	0	0	0.00005	0.0003	0.0006
Pinchin 1982	19	S	0	0	0	0.00042	0.0020	0.0030
CPSC 1987	45	R	0	0	0	0.00010	0	0.0020
McCrone 1991 (unpublished) schools	19	S	0	0	0.0002	0.00022	0.0005	0.0016
McCrone 1991 (unpublished) office	1	PC	—	—	—	0.00004	—	—

[a]Fibers greater than 5 μm.
[b]S = schools, PC = public and commercial buildings, R = residences.
[c]Only including buildings with asbestos.
From reference 47. Note that this is from "nonlitigation data."

scientific testimony on the exact nature of the risk. Distinguished physicians and pathologists have testified on both sides of many of these cases, the point at issue usually being the risk of low-level chrysotile exposure. In the United States, the need for quotable testimony, from scientific meetings, that favors one side or the other in such litigation, has led to "stacked" quasi-scientific meetings with speakers chosen to emphasize one side of the argument. In the recent Health Effects Institute report on asbestos (47), one table is headed, "Distribution of Building Average Airborne Asbestos Concentrations for Nonlitigation Data by Study," eloquent evidence of the role of the courts (see table 2.6). Asbestos is the dominant example among the five hazards under discussion in which extensive litigation has occurred. Its implications will be discussed later.

As I have noted elsewhere, much of the present confusion is attributable to the fact that different opinions can be legitimately held on the basis of the current evidence (48). There is no sign that the problem of asbestos-related disease has reached its peak. The hospital discharge rates for asbestosis for white males in New Jersey has risen from about 30 per 100,000 per year in 1979 to more than 150 per year in men over the age of 75 in 1986, and the rate does not appear to be flattening (see figure 2.8) (4). A recent paper from the Netherlands (50) describes the course of understanding the asbestos risk in that country. It is of interest that the rate of dissemination of knowledge and legislative action have both varied among countries in the free world.

The scientific basis for the present controversy can be briefly summarized as follows:

1. Current risk estimates are inevitably based on extrapolations from earlier epidemiological data for various occupations; there is considerable doubt as to the reliability of the exposure estimates that underlie these. Table 2.7, from the Health Effects Institute report, shows computed risks from environmental exposures; it is preceded by a note of three factors that are responsible for uncertainty. These are: (a) the uncertainty of historical occupational exposure data, from which low dose risks are extrapolated; (b) uncertainty about present levels of exposure to asbestos within buildings; and (c) uncertainty about the comparability of different methods of measuring airborne asbestos fibers.

2. Although mesothelioma is probably dose-response related,

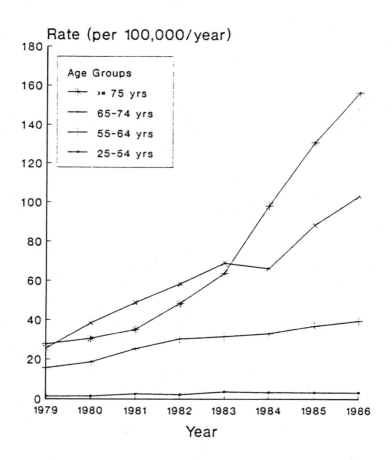

Figure 2.8. Annual age-specific discharge rates of asbestosis among white males in New Jersey, 1979–1986. Data from reference 49. Note that the hospital discharge rates for asbestosis in New Jersey have not yet started to fall.

about one-third of current cases have no known asbestos exposure (51). Huncharek (52) has recently summarized the evidence concerning the exposures to asbestos in cases of mesothelioma; the occupations of twenty-four men and sixteen women with mesothelioma—who had had no asbestos-related jobs or self-reported exposures—varied greatly. As the disease has a very long latent period (about thirty-three years in one series of cases), it may be questioned whether any possible impact from environmental exposure would now be visible. As noted above, the incidence of mesothelioma in the Netherlands is still rising.

3. Different types of asbestos fibers are known to disappear from

Table 2.7. Estimated Lifetime Cancer Risks for Different Scenarios of
Exposure to Airborne Asbestos Fibers[a]

Conditions	Premature Cancer Deaths (Lifetime Risks) per Million Exposed Persons
Lifetime, continuous outdoor exposure	
• 0.00001 f/mL from birth (rural)	4
• 0.0001 f/mL from birth (high urban)	40
Exposure in a school containing ACM, from age 5 to 18 years (180 days/year, 5 hours/day)	
• 0.0005 f/mL (average)[b]	6
• 0.005 f/mL (high)[b]	60
Exposure in a public building containing ACM age 25 to 45 years (240 days/year, 8 hours/day)	
• 0.0002 f/mL (average)[b]	4
• 0.002 f/mL (high)[b]	40
Occupational exposure from age 25 to 45	
• 0.1 f/mL (current occupational levels)[c]	2,000
• 10 f/mL (historical industrial exposures)	200,000

[a]This table represents the combined risk (average for males and females) estimated for lung cancer and mesothelioma for building occupants exposed to airborne asbestos fibers under the circumstances specified. These estimates should be interpreted with caution because of the reservations concerning the reliability of the estimates of average levels and of the risk assessment models summarized in Chapter 8.

[b]The "average" levels for the sampled schools and buildings represent the means of building averages for the buildings reviewed herein (Figure 1.1). The "high" levels for schools and public buildings, shown as 10 times the average, are approximately equal to the average airborne levels of asbestos recorded in approximately 5 percent of schools and buildings with asbestos-containing materials (ACM) (see Chapters 4 and 8). If the single highest sample value were excluded from calculation of the average indoor asbestos concentration in public and commercial buildings, the average value is reduced from 0.00021 to 0.00008 f/mL, and the lifetime risk is approximately halved.

[c]The concentration shown (0.1 f/mL) represents the permissible exposure limit (PEL) proposed by the U.S. Occupational Safety and Health Administration. Actual worker exposure, expected to be lower, will depend on a variety of factors including work practices, and use and efficiency of respiratory protective equipment.

From reference 47.

the lung at different rates. Chrysotile is cleared the fastest (53), and the more dangerous amphiboles, such as amosite and crocidolite, which are thought to lead to mesothelioma at lower exposures, are cleared much more slowly (54). This means that estimates of the numbers of residual fibers in the lung at autopsy may be unreliable guides to exposures.

4. The lungs of city dwellers (in Vancouver, for example) currently contain up to 40 million asbestos fibers (55). Churg, commenting recently on this finding (56), noted, "Yet despite this fiber burden, no epidemiological evidence exists to suggest that the general population

Table 2.8. Comparison of Lung Cancer Risks Estimated by Various Groups or Individuals from Studies of Asbestos-Exposed Workers[a]

| Study | Percent Increase in Lung Cancer Per f-y/mL of Exposure ($100 \times K_L$) | | | | |
	EPA[b]	CPSC[c]	NRC[d]	Ontario Royal Commission[e]	HSC[f]
Dement et al. (1983b)	2.8	2.3	5.3	4.2	
McDonald et al. (1983a)	2.5				1.25
Peto et al. (1985)[g]	1.1	1.0	0.8	1.0	0.54
McDonald et al. (1983b)	1.4				
Berry and Newhouse (1983)	0.058	0.06		0.058	
McDonald et al. (1984)	0.010				
McDonald et al. (1980)	0.06	0.06	0.06	0.020–0.046	
Nicholson et al. (1979)	0.17	0.12	0.15		
Rubino et al. (1979)	0.075	0.17			
Seidman (1984)	4.3	6.8[h]	9.1[h]		
Selikoff et al. (1979)	0.75	1.0	1.7	1.0	
Henderson and Enterline (1979)	0.49	0.50	0.3	0.069	
Weill et al. (1979)	0.53	0.31			
Finkelstein (1983)	6.7	4.8		4.2[i]	
Newhouse and Berry (1979)					
Males			1.3		
Females			8.4		
Values used for risk extrapolation	1.0	0.3–3.0	2.0	0.02–4.2	1.0

[a]Adapted from Nicholson (1986).

[b]U.S. Environmental Protection Agency (Nicholson 1986).

[c]U.S. Consumer Product Safety Commission (1983).

[d]National Research Council (1984).

[e]Ontario Royal Commission (1984).

[f]U.K. Health and Safety Commission (Doll and Peto 1985).

[g]Earlier reviews cited Peto (1978) or Peto (1980), and some noted that all men employed after 1951 suffered a higher dose-specific risk ($100 \times K_L = 1.5$).

[h]Data from Seidman and colleagues (1979).

[i]Unpublished data supplied to the Commission.

From reference 47. Note the ranges of risk estimates. In the case of asbestos, there is probably only a small error in outcome measurement; the uncertainty lies in estimates of past exposure.

suffers from any type of asbestos related disease." With a hazard apparently now so widely disseminated, how could one evaluate its contribution to the incidence of lung cancer?

These issues indicate that it is largely scientific uncertainty, together with the problem of extrapolating from high to low exposures, that feeds the present highly litigous environment. The consequences of this will be examined in Chapter 4.

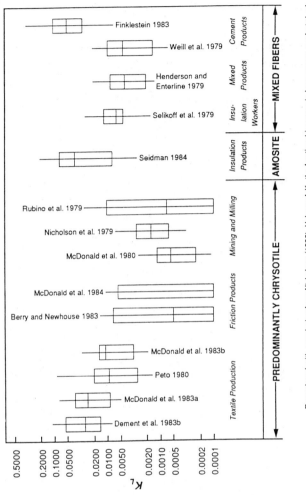

Reproduced with permission from Nicholson (1986). Values of K_L, the fractional increase in lung cancer per f·y/mL of exposure in 14 asbestos exposed cohorts. The open bar reflects the estimated 95 percent confidence limits associated with measures of response. The line represents the uncertainties associated with measures of exposure, generally plus or minus a factor of two. For discussion of uncertainties associated with exposure assessment and response measure, see text.

Figure 2.9. The risk of lung cancer in different occupations and with different fibers. From reference 47. Note the generally higher levels of risk in secondary industries compared to those in mining and milling of asbestos.

Therefore, in the case of asbestos, current controversy involves the risk of long-term, low-level exposures; biological plausibility is not an issue; there are differences of opinion on the relative risks of different fiber types; and the debate is complicated by problems of exposure assessment, different rates of fiber clearance from the lung, and the long latent period before effects appear. In the United States, the legal process has subsumed scientific discussion of these problems, and media interest is sporadic. Asbestos companies, actively backed in Canada by the government, have been pushing sales of the mineral in the Third World. It is exceedingly unlikely that the safe use of asbestos can be guaranteed in these countries, though the industry asserts that this is the case. In 1987, I published an editorial (57) that raised the question of whether the medical profession in Canada should consider itself responsible for the uncontrolled export of such dangerous material to the Third World, but to this date no effective action has been taken by any government agency or professional organization with respect to it.

Lead

Articles on lead commonly begin with the observation that the hazards of lead mining were known to the Romans. Indeed, some historians have regarded lead poisoning as an important factor contributing to the decline of the Roman Empire. In most modern cases, questions of lead poisoning have arisen in connection with emissions from a local smelter or battery recovery plant. The tortuous process of inquiry, political responsibility, and confused scientific evidence in the case of a small plant in Toronto has been excellently documented by Salter (58). In Trail, British Columbia, the long-term operation of a large smelter has led to increased lead in the soil in the adjacent town and to raised blood lead levels in the residents (59).

However, the widespread use of lead in gasoline was responsible for dissemination of this mineral, even into the Greenland ice cap (see figure 2.10; 60). The symptoms of acute lead poisoning in adults and in children were generally recognized before 1939. What has transformed the discussion is that beginning in 1943, epidemiological data indicate that even at very low levels the blood lead in children is related to behavioral changes and a lowering of IQ. This important

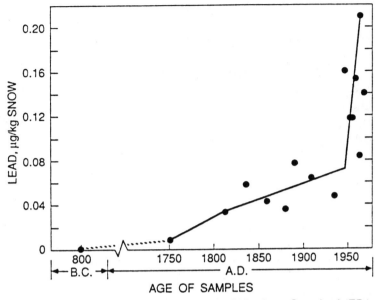

Lead concentration, profile in snow strata of Northern Greenland (EPA, 1986).

Figure 2.10. Lead concentration profile in Greenland snow strata, A.D. 1750 to A.D. 1970. From reference 60. The increase in lead in the snow strata of Greenland is a consequence of its wide dispersal in fine particulate form in gasoline.

controversy has recently been summarized in a collected series of papers that provide an excellent review of the data from different countries (61):

1. Needleman, who pioneered the first large studies relating lead level in deciduous teeth or blood level to behavioral and intelligence parameters, has recently summarized twenty-four studies of this type (62). The regression coefficients for lead levels against IQ were negative in eleven of the twelve studies in which it was calculated. This means that the higher the blood lead, the larger is the decrement from the predicted IQ.

2. In 1986, a small commission convened by the Royal Society of Canada (63) at the request of the government, heard evidence relating to lead and its effects. The summary and conclusions noted:

8. Much controversy persists concerning the nature of the relationship between blood lead and neuropsychological effects in children. Two major problems are:

• the difficulty in determining the relative contributions of lead and socio-demographic factors to neuropsychological functions of children.

• the difficulties in interpretation arising from the smallness of the effects commonly attributed to lead at the blood lead levels encountered among children. Current studies being conducted prospectively have yet to confirm the observations reported in earlier studies. However, the consistency of the direction of the association, even after statistical adjustment for confounding variables, suggests that the effect is indeed real, though small.

9. Other effects on the central nervous system have been suggested by neurophysiological studies of the central nervous system in children. These studies have yielded conflicting results that are hard to interpret. The Commission considers them to be still experimental.

The commission nevertheless recommended that lead should be removed from gasoline. The 1987 report to the Canadian Environmental Assessment Research Council (64) reviewed the epidemiological data and argued that earlier risk estimates had underestimated the totality of risks from exposure to lead.

2. The results from a European multicenter study (65) conducted in Bulgaria, Denmark, Greece, Hungary, Italy, Rumania, West Germany, and Yugoslavia, and involving 1879 children whose blood lead levels varied between 5 and 60 micrograms/100 ml, concluded that "there are detectable exposure-related neurobehavioral effects in school age children." This was published in 1990.

3. A 1988 British Medical Research Council (MRC) advisory committee (66) review of the data then available concluded, "While the observed statistical associations detailed in this review are consistent with the hypothesis that low-level lead exposure has a small negative effect on the performance of children in ability and attainment tests, the limitations of epidemiological studies in drawing causal inferences are such that it is not possible to conclude that exposure to lead at

current urban levels is definitely harmful." This paragraph is discussed in detail later.

4. A recent U.S. National Academy of Sciences report on neurotoxicology (67) used lead to illustrate the importance of a minor (5 percent) downward shift in mean IQ score (figure 2.11). In a population of 100 million children, such a change results in a fall in the number of individuals with an IQ greater than 130 from 2.3 million to 990,000. Those scoring less than 70 rise correspondingly in numbers from 990,000 to 2.3 million. Figure 2.12 shows an illustration of the relationship between umbilical cord lead and an index of mental development.

The contemporary argument lies partly in the interpretation of the epidemiological data in terms of causality (discussed later), and partly in the variability of indices of childhood behavior, attention span, and IQ measurements. In the recent volume on lead (68), Needleman and Beringer contributed a paper entitled "Type II Fallacies in the Study of Childhood Exposure to Lead at Low Dose: A Critical and Quantitative Review." They noted, "Making causal connections in the real world is not a pure, value-free enterprise."

> It seems clear that differences in style exist among investigators and interpreters of the same data base. These stylistic, value-laden differences in interpreting the data seem to be rather stable traits.

A Type II error is to deny a causal link when it is later shown to exist (see page 65).

The many pathways of lead exposure in children are shown in figure 2.13 (69). For some years the industry interested in keeping lead in gasoline argued that airborne lead from vehicles was such a minor component of the lead intake of children that its elimination would have little effect on blood levels. However, the reduction of lead in gasoline in the United States has been closely paralleled by a remarkable fall in the blood lead of children, which unquestionably indicates that automobile-derived lead was of far greater importance than had been realized (see figure 2.14).

Although lead levels in blood and deciduous teeth are useful biomarkers of lead exposure, they are not without limitations. Blood lead

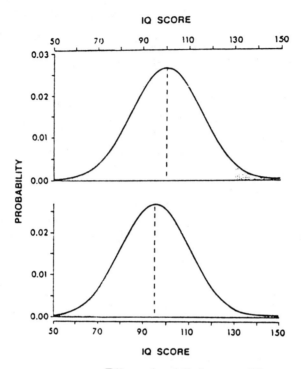

Effect of a shift in mean IQ score on the population distribution. The top figure represents a theoretical population distribution of IQ scores with a mean of 100 and a standard deviation of 15. In a population of 100 million, 2.3 million (stippled area) will score above 130. The bottom figure represents distribution of intelligence-test scores with a shift of 5%, yielding a mean of 95. Here, the number of individuals scoring above 130 falls to 990 thousand, with a corresponding inflation of those scoring below 70. Source: Weiss (1990).

Figure 2.11. Effect of a 5 percent mean shift in IQ in a population of 100 million. From reference 67. A shift in mean IQ score of 5 percent in a large population has major implications in terms of changes at either end of the distribution curve.

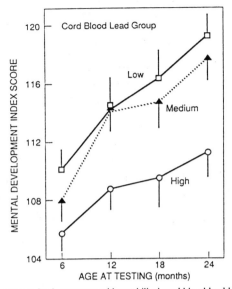

Prenatal exposure to lead, as measured by umbilical cord blood lead levels vs early mental development index. Low is ≤3 μg/dl, medium is 6.7 μg/dl, and high is ≥10 μg/dl (Bellinger *et al.*, 1987).

Figure 2.12. Prenatal lead exposure vs. mental development. From reference 67. A more specific index of mental development in children shows significant depression in relation to umbilical cord levels greater than 10 micrograms/ml.

is believed to have a half-life of about thirty-six days; therefore a single observation cannot be taken as representative of past exposure. New methods of noninvasive detection of the lead level in bone may prove useful in adults, but may be difficult to interpret in growing children.

There has been remarkably little public concern expressed at the hazard represented by lead in gasoline. There do not appear to be any major public health societies that have taken up the issue, though in the United States there is an Alliance to End Childhood Lead Poisoning. In the United States, the debate before legislators was carried out between scientists representing industry, on the one hand, and those with a long interest in the mineral and its adverse health effects on the other. This debate received little significant media coverage. Unlike the case of asbestos, the lead issue has not been the subject of detailed litigation, and no courts have had to rule on the likelihood of a raised

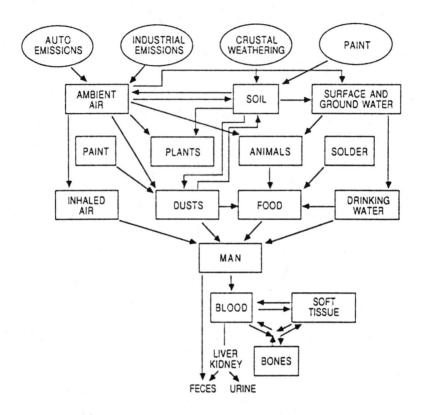

Figure 2.13. Pathways of lead exposure. From reference 69. There was much uncertainty as to which route of exposure might be dominant in the case of children, but the fall in blood lead levels that accompanied the decline in lead use in gasoline in the United States (see figure 2.14) indicated that direct inhalation or indirect contact with automobile lead must have been a dominant pathway.

blood lead level being a cause of mental retardation in an individual case. Recently, the lead industry has apparently decided to mount a campaign questioning the integrity of the epidemiologists who have studied its effects in children.

Before the decision was made to remove lead from gasoline, the U.S. Environmental Protection Agency (EPA) summarized the adverse health effects of lead, particularly emphasizing the relationship between blood lead levels and hypertension that had been found in a random sample of men in a national survey. The epidemiological data on children were noted, but no attempt was made to base a cost/

LEAD AND HUMAN HEALTH

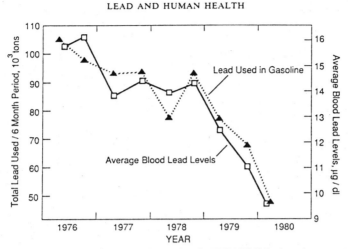

Parallel decreases in blood lead values observed in the NHANES II Study and amounts of lead used in gasoline during 1976–1980 (EPA, 1986).

Figure 2.14. Decreases in blood lead and use of lead in gasoline in the United States from 1976 to 1980. From reference 69. The remarkable concomitant fall in blood lead values—in a subset of a 50,000-person random sample in the United States—with the reduction of lead in gasoline indicates the dominance of this source in general public exposure to the metal.

benefit analysis on them. At the same time, the automobile industry concluded that the newly required reductions in automobile emissions, particularly of hydrocarbons, necessitated the use of a catalytic converter on the exhaust system. This equipment could only be used if the gasoline was lead free. There was, therefore, a conjunction between these two aspects of lead, and both undoubtedly played a part in the decision to reduce its use in gasoline. It does not seem possible to answer the question of whether a decision based on health data alone would have been to discontinue the use of lead in gasoline. By 1985, however, the adverse health effects of lead had been more clearly delineated, and the resulting health costs were computed at that time by the EPA. These considerations played a role in the decision to remove lead altogether from gasoline.

The lead controversy therefore involves both the routes of uptake and the importance of shifts in the measured IQ in groups of children; there are special aspects in relation to biological plausibility; and there is no significant public pressure group in any jurisdiction, and little media interest. The belief in the importance of removing lead from gasoline was early and strong in the United States, but later and reluctant in the case of Canada and Britain. This reluctance is difficult to explain. However, one may note that in the section on lead in the World Health Organization publication *Air Quality Guidelines for Europe* (70), published in 1987, there seems to be some confusion over the routes of intake of lead in children, since the report does not recognize that road dust may contain lead from gasoline. The report (on page 256) concluded that in children "the contribution of direct inhalation to total lead absorption is smaller than in adults (approximately 6% only). Most of the absorbed dose can be accounted for by other pathways, mainly food." This seems to have been the reasoning that underlay the reluctance of British experts to believe that lead in gasoline was important. The concomitant fall in blood lead levels with reduction of the lead in gasoline shown in figure 2.14 indicates that lead in gasoline must be a major factor in determining contemporary blood lead levels.

Lead in all its forms represents a signficant hazard in the developing world. According to data published by the World Bank, Karachi, Pakistan, now has the highest lead content of gasoline of any major city. The impact of this on the neurobehavioral development of the children there can only be imagined.

Electromagnetic Fields

In figure 2.15 are shown the various wavelengths and energies of electromagnetic fields (EMF) and where these fit into the energy spectrum (71). The fields that may be induced in such a complex structure as the human body are extremely variable and depend on a variety of factors too detailed for the present discussion. These considerations underlie the difficulty of knowing how to assess exposure.

In 1979, Wertheimer and Leeper (72) published a paper in the *American Journal of Epidemiology* in which they reported finding a significant association between leukemia in children and the wiring configuration of the electrical distribution lines supplying the houses in Denver in which the children were living. The wiring configuration was thought to be a surrogate for the EMF exposure to which the children had been subjected. The authors wrote a very cautious interpretation of their data. In table 2.1, I have dated the initial public concern about

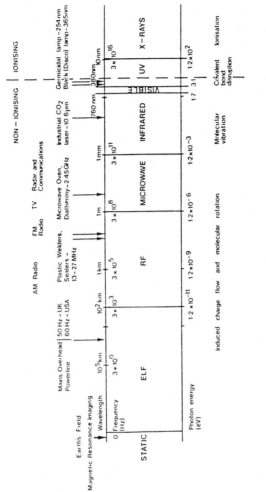

Figure 2.15. The electromagnetic spectrum. From reference 71. The second arrow from the left indicates the energy range of EMF exposures to overhead power lines.

this risk to 1986, since by that date there had been a number of supporting studies. In 1982, it was first suggested that men and women working in occupations that might increase their exposure to electromagnetic fields faced an increased risk of various forms of cancer. By 1990, the EPA had issued a draft report entitled *Evaluation of the Potential Carcinogenicity of Electromagnetic Fields* (73). This report engendered so much heated reaction that a subcommittee of the EPA's Science Advisory Board was put together to review it and to make recommendations. The subcommittee reported in December 1991 (74), and required a full rewrite of the literature review and its intepretation.

The present status of this issue is one of exceptional interest, as will be evident from the following observations.

1. The visual presentations of risk ratios for electrical workers prepared by Theriault (75; see figures 2.16 and 2.17) indicate a clear preponderance of studies with risk ratios greater than 1, and in some cases as high as 2.8. Theriault points out that case-control studies have generally given a positive result, but cohort studies have been uniformly negative. This is unexplained.

2. In the case of childhood leukemia, two recent studies, one in Denver and another in California, have confirmed Wertheimer and Leeper's original observation. The recently published study by London and Peters and their colleagues in Los Angeles (76) analyzed 219 cases of leukemia in children and compared them to 232 controls. Measurements of magnetic and electrical fields were made in the homes of 164 of the cases and 144 of the controls; wiring configuration was noted in 219 cases and 109 controls. The authors reported an odds ratio of 2.15 (95 percent confidence limits 1.08–4.28) for very high, relative to very low, current and ground configuration data (see table 2.9). (An odds ratio of 2 means that a risk is doubled. The confidence limits define the possible lower and upper limits to the incurred risk, one indicating no increase, and 4.0, for example, indicating a fourfold increase.) There was no association with the measured electromagnetic fields in the child's home. The cases were more likely than the controls to report use of several appliances in the home that produce high electric and magnetic fields.

This study therefore confirmed the Denver data of Wertheimer and Leeper showing a significant association between wiring configuration and leukemia risk. The authors noted,

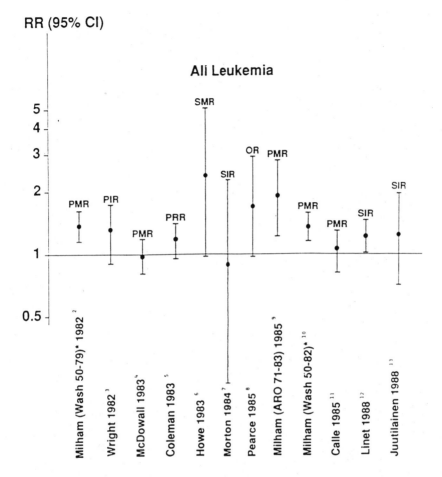

Figure 2.16. Leukemia risks among electrical workers. From reference 75. Note that two studies showed a relative risk of less than one, and, in a further six, the lower level of the 95 percent confidence limits is below one. In view of the absence of precise exposure data, the balance of the data might be taken to indicate a probable relationship.

Unfortunately, there is little known about the etiology of childhood cancer, and therefore, confounding by a factor not known to be a disease risk is possible. Yet such a factor would need to be strongly associated with risk or extremely tightly correlated with wiring configuration classification to have produced the odds ratio in our study and others.

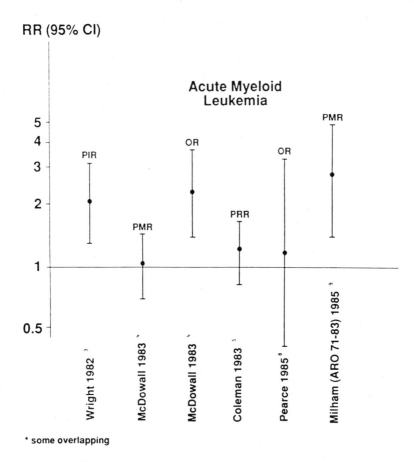

RR (95% CI)

Acute Myeloid
Leukemia

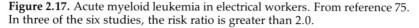

* some overlapping

Figure 2.17. Acute myeloid leukemia in electrical workers. From reference 75. In three of the six studies, the risk ratio is greater than 2.0.

This study involved the most detailed attempt to exclude other confounders that one can imagine. The confirmation of the original Denver data in another city and in a larger sample surely indicates that the epidemiological data cannot be dismissed.

3. Recently, an excess of breast cancers in men (which are rare tumors) occupationally exposed to EMF has been reported. This might be linked to changes in melatonin secretion. Theriault has recently written (75):

> It has been proposed recently that the mechanism by which EMF may participate in the development of cancer

Table 2.9. Leukemia Risk in Relation to Denver Wertheimer-Leeper Wiring Configuration Classification, Los Angeles County, California, 1980–1987

Exposure category*	Cases	Controls	OR†	95% CI†	p for trend
Underground	11	11			
Very low	20	27	1.00‡		
Ordinary low	58	75	0.95	0.53–1.69	
Ordinary high	80	68	1.44	0.81–2.56	
Very high	42	24	2.15	1.08–4.26	
					0.008 (4 categories)
					0.012 (all 5 categories)

statistically significant

*Mixed overhead/underground removed (eight cases and two controls).

†OR, odds ratio; CI, confidence interval.

‡Reference category is underground and very low combined. Wiring configuration classification for the residence lived in the longest was used.

From reference 76. Data from the Los Angeles study of childhood leukemia confirming the earlier finding of Wertheimer and Leeper in Denver.

in men is the decrease in melatonin hormone in blood. Melatonin is known to influence the development of hormone sensitive cancers in animals. . . . Recent findings of excesses of male breast cancer among electrical workers and of excess of skin melanoma in cohorts of telecommunications, electrical and electronic workers may be a serious indication that EMF may indeed contribute to the development of cancer through the decreased melatonin pathway.

4. Hutchison (77) considered that central nervous system cancer in children represented the strongest association with residential exposure to EMF.

5. The Nonionizing Electric and Magnetic Fields Subcommittee of the EPA Science Advisory Board (74) convened to review the draft report on potential carcinogenicity, concluded:

Some epidemiological evidence is suggestive of an association between surrogate measurements of magnetic field exposure and certain cancer outcomes. In such studies, the existence of confounders is always a possibility, but since no common confounder has yet been identified, the existing evidence cannot be dismissed.

6. The most relevant biological data on the effects of electromagnetic fields seem to be those indicating some interference with the secretion of melatonin, a hormone produced by the pineal gland that has something to do with the circadian rhythm but that in addition may inhibit tumor growth or formation. Physicists have argued that EMF at 60 hertz cannot affect individual cells, but they concede that whole glands or neural networks might be affected. This would explain why radar confuses migrating birds, and why some fish seem capable of detecting very low energy electromagnetic fields. However, the biological plausibility for a direct carcinogenic effect in the human cannot be said to be strong.

7. The 1992 British Medical Research Council Report (71), after an exhaustive and excellently written review of the present status of the whole field (including the recent Los Angeles study), came to a number of conclusions:

> The experimental findings are, unfortunately, not very helpful. It cannot be concluded either that the electromagnetic fields have no effect on the physiology of cells, even if the fields are weak, or that they produce effects that would, in other circumstances, be regarded as suggestive of potential carcinogenicity.
>
> The results of some whole animal and cellular studies suggest the possibility that electromagnetic fields might act as co-carcinogens or tumour promoters but, taken overall, the data are inconclusive.

In relation to cancer in children:

> The results have been variable, but, taken at face value, they appear to provide some weak evidence in support of the postulated association which is less weak for brain cancer than for leukemia and less weak when exposure is estimated from the local "wire configurations" than from proximity to sources of electromagnetic fields or from measurements in the home.
>
> This evidence is, however, difficult to accept as the methodology of the most important studies failed to obtain sets of control data that could be confidently regarded as repre-

sentative of the populations from which the affected children were drawn. The major positive results may in consequence be artefacts of the method of enquiry. In summary, the epidemiological findings that have been reviewed provide no firm evidence of the existence of a carcinogenic hazard from exposure of paternal gonads, the fetus, children, or adults to the extremely low frequency electromagnetic fields that might be associated with residence near major sources of electricity supply, the use of electrical appliances, or work in the electrical, electronic, and telecommunications industries.

The main criticism of the Los Angeles study was directed at the method of selecting the controls and in the uncertainty over whether wiring configuration actually represented any significant difference in electromagnetic exposure. Sir Richard Doll (the chair of the committee) is quoted later as saying, "It is, we suggest, important that more research is carried out to clarify as soon as possible whether extremely low frequency magnetic fields in the home and at work are capable of causing cancer." This report therefore was significantly more negative in relation to the existing epidemiological data than was the report of the subcommittee of the EPA's Science Advisory Board or the reports by Hutchison and Theriault referred to above. One might wonder why it is important that more research be carried out on the question if the present epidemiological data can be dismissed as nonsubstantive.

8. Two recent reports, contained in manuscripts not yet published in the open literature, are not reassuring. In a Swedish case-control study of people who had lived for at least one year within 300 meters of a 200 or 400 kilovolt transmission line (78), an increased relative risk of 2.7 for childhood leukemia was found. In another large Swedish study of workers occupationally exposed to electromagnetic fields (79), a significant excess of chronic lymphatic leukemia was found. It was not considered that confounding by exposure to solvents or benzene could have occurred. Though these two studies have not yet appeared in the scientific literature, they will both reinforce previous data when they are published.

9. There is no doubt that difficulties in measuring exposure, or in knowing what aspect of exposure might be important (e.g., mean levels, transients, lifetime averages) not only make interpretation of the

epidemiological data difficult, but also cause problems in designing appropriate animal studies. All are agreed that refinement of exposure data, particularly in those occupationally exposed to electromagnetic fields, is of first importance. It must be remembered that exposure misclassification is likely to have the effect of weakening a demonstrated relationship. Indeed, one can view the epidemiological data and remark that it is astonishing that any relationship should have been found in view of the obvious and serious weakness of exposure classification.

There has been considerable public interest in this issue. A recent book (80) has summarized various enquiry processes and events in relation to electromagnetic fields; the author alleges a major conspiracy in the scientific community to prevent the truth being known. In many areas, there have been hearings and inquiries on the location of high-voltage power transmission lines, and in British Columbia the hydroelectric authority has agreed to purchase, at fair price, houses that lie very close to necessary new transmission lines. Some scientists who have long been involved with electromagnetic fields have urged a policy of "prudent avoidance" until the facts become better established. Major new research initiatives to clarify animal effects, and to extend the epidemiological observations, have been launched. New technologies are being developed to permit better exposure evaluation. All of these steps should be useful in resolving the present dilemma. It should be noted that the electric blanket manufacturing industry, once it had been shown that the blankets were capable of generating strong magnetic fields, redesigned them, with the result that modern blankets now deliver a negligible dose.

The electric generating industry has financed efforts to question the validity of the epidemiological data, but these have not included overt attempts to discredit the epidemiologists who have conducted such studies.

Electromagnetic field effects pose, in acute form, the problem of interpreting epidemiological associations when there is little biological plausibility and no demonstrated dose-response relationship. This problem receives more discussion in the next chapter.

In the case of electromagnetic fields, therefore, the reason for concern is based entirely on the epidemiological evidence; there are very difficult problems in exposure assessment; biological plausibility is a major problem; there is much media interest; and significant indus-

good

trial lobbies are involved. The question of whether leukemia is a multifactorial disease, with EMF exposure being one factor, cannot yet be settled.

Summary

This brief perspective on the five hazards I have chosen to discuss permits some preliminary generalizations.

As far as epidemiological studies are concerned, in the case of cigarettes the overwhelming associative evidence is accepted as indicating a causal link to lung cancer and emphysema. There is basic biological plausibility, a clearly demonstrated dose-response relationship to risk, and a very large number of studies in different countries that confirm the strong associative relationship. Cigarette smoking is also recognized as one risk factor in the multifactorial nature of heart disease.

In the case of air pollution, different types of epidemiological studies are used to describe adverse effects; each of these has strengths and weaknesses, as noted in the next chapter. Only when a major single episode occurs, as in London in 1952 or in Donora in 1948, is the evidence so strong that the causal link cannot be disputed. In more general cases, cross-sectional studies or time-series analyses require detailed discussion and replication before it is reasonable to infer a causal relationship and before general confounders can be excluded. For some pollutants, such as ozone, there is a strong basis of biological plausibility; in the case of particulate pollution or the possible effects of very low exposures to sulfur dioxide, no biological mechanisms are yet known to explain the associations that have been described. In the case of particles less than 10 microns in size, the regression against mortality on a daily basis is so strong, and has been demonstrated to apply in cities so different in climate and population, that there are strong grounds for concluding that the relationship is causal, even in the absence of any known biological mechanism.

disagree

The general relationships of asbestos to lung cancer and mesothelioma have been well established. The more difficult questions of risk in relation to fiber type, and of defining general levels of public exposure, remain to be fully elucidated. Much of the present controversy revolves around these questions.

good

Epidemiological studies in relation to lead, although reasonably comprehensive and almost unanimous in relation to the hazard it represents for young children, still occasion different interpretations. Some take the position that the effect is too small to be of consequence; others disagree.

The epidemiological data about electromagnetic field exposure tend to point in the same direction, but their interpretation is made difficult by the lack of any dose-response relationship and by very weak biological plausibility. No common confounder in all the studies has been identified.

The general questions raised by epidemiological studies are dealt with in detail in the next chapter. It is clear, from four of the five hazards discussed, that the interpretation of epidemiological data is central to understanding how each of them should be approached. Only in the case of cigarettes is the data complete, though of course this was not the case when the first studies were published.

Public involvement in these five hazards has varied from intense, in the case of cigarettes and electromagnetic fields, to episodic in the case of air pollution, to surprisingly almost absent in relation to lead. Environmental exposure to asbestos, though this has received intermittent attention centering around publicized litigation, in general has not become a major public issue.

The role of the media generally reflects the level of public concern (indeed it is difficult to separate these two aspects). The media also have the effect of focusing public attention on an issue, and may be said to stimulate public concern. In the case of cigarettes, the printed media were initially inhibited by the threat of withdrawal of cigarette advertising, which is an important source of revenue. Such publications as the original U.S. Surgeon General's report and subsequent yearly follow-up reports have subsequently ensured wide media coverage. Surveys indicate that most members of the public in the United States are now aware of the dangers of cigarette smoking. The decline in smoking, though slow to start, may be attributed to government intervention based on public concern. It is interesting that there was a gap of several years between the first publication of summaries of the epidemiological data (as in the Surgeon General's report of 1963) and the development of public interest groups to represent the interests of nonsmokers. These groups became much more active after the effect of passive smoke inhalation began to be publicized.

In some regions, and in relation to some types of air pollution, the media have played an important role. This was especially true in relation to the 1952 London episode, when media pressure drove a reluctant government to set up a committee to study the question. In Los Angeles, and in the question of acid rain in the northeastern United States and Canada, the media have played an important role in public education.

Media attention to asbestos has been confined to publicizing individual cases of mesothelioma or lung cancer in those who have been occupationally exposed. This publicity undoubtedly has had an effect on juries charged with the assessment of responsibility and the awarding of damages. There has been little general media coverage of the risks that may follow general environmental exposure to asbestos.

It is surprising that very little public discussion has taken place about the question of the effects of lead at low-level exposures. This may be because individual cases cannot be highlighted. The point will be made in the next chapter that it is one thing to say that a community's exposure to lead is too high and should be reduced, and quite another to tell parents that the low IQ of their child has been caused by their living close to a main traffic artery.

The media have been very much involved in the question of electromagnetic fields. Wherever effects have been attributed to high-tension transmission lines or to the location of a transformer station at the end of the road, the media have been willing to publicize the public concern aroused. As noted later, this coverage has generally not been sophisticated. The authors of the most recent study of electromagnetic fields and childhood leukemia (76) were blamed for a newspaper's apparently biased coverage of their paper. In a letter to the editor of the *American Journal of Epidemiology* in which their study had been published, they observed:

> Our paper was written for the scientific literature, not the public media. We assumed that those seriously interested in the issue would read the entire paper. There is limited space in an abstract, and it is impossible to word it to avoid all possible opportunities for the media to misrepresent the findings. Furthermore, very few of the reporters who contacted us had even read the abstract. We made every at-

tempt to clarify the results in our dealings with the media and have come to the conclusion that the media presentation is largely beyond our control.

In the case of asbestos, the discussion of the interpretation of existing data has been carried on almost entirely in relation to litigation. The same is true to a lesser extent in relation to electromagnetic fields. The involvement of courts and individual law firms has had various consequences that have not been evident in relation to the other hazards.

As might be expected, the role of industry and industrial consortia has been defensive. Such groups command enormous financial potential, not just that derived from the sale of their products, but also from the power given them over governments by virtue of taxation income, and, in the case of tobacco, over the media by virtue of advertising revenue.

Before any general conclusions can be reached in relation to these five hazards and the lessons to be drawn from them, there are six issues that require detailed discussion. These are the subject of the next chapter.

3

Mandated Science: Major Issues in Health and Public Policy

In her text with this title (58), Salter describes "mandated science" as involving the relationship of science, values, and public policy, and illustrates this by a Venn diagram (see figure 3.1). This provides a useful framework for the discussion of the interrelationships involved.

Over the period of the present review, covering approximately the past forty years, scientists have generally become conscious of the importance of distinguishing between their statements that are based solely on a description of the scientific data, and other judgments they may make, which are just that. They have, in general, learned the necessity of being sensitive to the difference between their opinion on an issue and an analysis of the available data that is not weighted by value judgment. It is evident that an inference of causality from a demonstrated association requires a judgment; it is important to treat it as such.

A number of authors have written on the intersection between science and values. The valuable volume by Loren Graham (81), written in 1981, provides an excellent starting point. A recent interesting discussion of the relationship between values and judgments particularly relevant to environmental concerns is that by Steensberg (82) in his analysis of environmental decision making in Denmark.

It is important to recognize that both policy decisions, such as removing lead from gasoline or protecting the public from high-tension transmission lines or from ozone exposure, and all discussions of standard setting take place within the area between "values" and "science." Such discussions require, first, agreement as to what

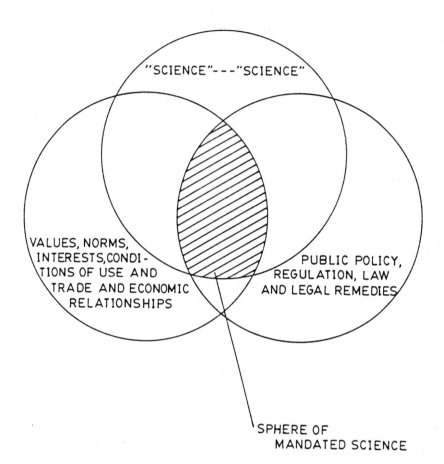

Figure 3.1. "Mandated Science." From reference 58. Note that "mandated science" exists in the overlapping zone between "science," "policy and regulation," and "values." Many scientists find this position an uncomfortable one.

the scientific data say and the existence of a causal relationship; and, second, statements of the "values" or economic considerations that underly the final decision. These must be made explicit and discussed on their own. What often happens is that the interpretation of the scientific data is skewed (in one direction or another) on the basis of (unstated) "values" held by the speaker.

Salter also addresses another important question when she writes:

> What seems to be true is that the problem of combining science and advocacy occurred when scientists and their

> work were being evaluated outside the scientific commu-
> nity and by non-scientists. It is this observation that leads
> us to identify the problem in the relationship between sci-
> ence and advocacy not in the conduct of the research but in
> its presentation to a non-scientific community.

This touches on the relationship between science and the law, discussed later.

What has happened in the past forty years is that "science" has
perforce moved out into the community. Certainly it has been central
to the issues of environmental epidemiology with which this text is
concerned. In discussing this background, Salter writes, "This
quandary—the increasing dependence upon science and technology
and an increasing concern or skepticism about the kind of answers
that science itself can provide—is the heart of the matter." It is for
this reason that the precise interpretation of environmental epidemiological data is central to these issues of environmental hazards.

There is another aspect to mandated science that has to do with the
implications of science that is not conducted as "free inquiry" but that
is conducted to elucidate some problem that has become important.
In this category are the controlled studies of the acute effects of air
pollutants, or the attempts to study the effects of lead or electromagnetic fields on animals. This type of science is directly concerned with
the setting of standards for the protection of public health; indeed,
Salter's text is subtitled *Science and Scientists in the Making of Standards*.
This question is discussed in Chapter 5.

Statistical Associations

In his history of statistics, subtitled *"The Measurement of Uncertainty
before 1900*, Stigler (83) notes that Yule's first use of a correlation coefficient (later refined by Karl Pearson) was in the study of characteristics
of the poor and criminal classes. Its use for this purpose was challenged by Pigou in written testimony before a Royal Commission on
the Poor Law. Pigou based his criticism on the possibility of an unmea-
sured "lurking variable" interfering with what Yule had suggested
was a causal relationship. Thus the argument concerning the meaning
and interpretation of a statistical association began right at the start of
its formulation.

The Pearson correlation coefficient (see table 2.2) is the simplest way of determining that a relationship between two variables is not a random distribution. A more sophisticated method involves the calculation of a regression coefficient (which may be shown to be statistically significant) between the two variables. Such coefficients, which relate relative incremental changes in the variables, are called "elasticities" by economists. When used in relation to air pollution data, as an example, these elasticities become changed to the form, "A 50 percent fall in the level of atmospheric sulphates would lead to a 15 percent reduction in hospital admissions for acute respiratory disease." Causality is assumed.

In most modern epidemiological work, the design of the study involves 1) data collection to account for all known variables; 2) correction of the basic data for these variables by filtering of one kind or another; and 3) the model's prediction of the relationship between the two variables of interest, such as the wiring configuration of houses and leukemia, or particulate pollution and mortality, or blood lead and IQ level. This application of logistic regression and modeling may become so complex that it is easy to lose sight of the fact that, at the end of it all, what is being assessed is the robustness of an association—that is, its ability to withstand the taking into account of other factors.

In some studies, such as the study of associations between atmospheric variables and hospital admissions, certain difficulties can be avoided by the design of the database rather than by later statistical manipulation of the data. Thus, in the case of the Ontario study (23), each summer can be considered separately to avoid long-term effects, or the respiratory admissions on a given day of the week can be compared only to the mean value for the same day of the week, and so on. Such preliminary treatment of the data avoids having long-term effects produce a spurious relationship, which is always a hazard of associative analysis.

With all environmental hazards, the existence of unidentified confounders is invariably a possibility. Cross-sectional comparisons of one population with another (such as symptom prevalence in children in a high-pollution region compared to children in a low-pollution region) are always complicated by other differences between the two populations—in this case in socioeconomic circumstances, in housing quality, in gas cooking, in maternal cigarette smoking, and in other

factors. These difficulties in cross-sectional comparisons make the lon-
gitudinal time-series studies—based on variations from day to day—
somewhat easier to interpret. These studies state that, in a given population, there is an association between one event, such as elevated
pollution, and another, such as hospital admissions or mortality. The
possible role of confounders is often misunderstood. When I submitted
my first paper on the air-pollution-to-hospital-admissions relationship
in southern Ontario, one reviewer objected that I had taken no account
of the cigarette smoking of the population. A moment's thought shows
that in this kind of study, this objection is irrelevant. This is because the
significant association is a time relationship between pollutant and
number of hospital admissions.

In the case of electromagnetic fields, the studies on the association
between home wiring configuration and childhood leukemia might be
affected if there was a chance association between wiring configuration of the house and its being adjacent to major traffic arteries. In the
occupationally exposed cohorts, exposure to organic chemicals or sol-
der in the course of electrical work might well occur but would not be
accounted for in the studies. Similarly, the association between blood
lead levels in children and their IQ has been dismissed on the
grounds that blood lead is possibly elevated in children in whom
some other factor is operative, such as low family income, and it is
this that drives the association. This possibility appears to have influenced the conclusions of the committee of the Royal Society of Canada that considered the issue.

Inferring Causality from Associations

It is clear that the problem of inferring causality from demonstrated
associations lies at the heart of the debates on the five hazards. This
question was first discussed in any detail in a series of articles in the
Journal of Chronic Diseases in 1959 and 1960 (see Labarthe and Stallone's
article in reference [84] for this). However, the problem of concluding
that causality underlies a demonstrated association was brought into
prominence in a presidential address by Sir Austin Bradford Hill (85) to
the Royal Society of Medicine in London in 1965. Hill had made many
distinguished contributions to statistical theory and practice. He did
not lay down specific or rigid "laws" that should govern this process,
but rather listed factors that he suggested were helpful in formulating a

judgment that the associations might be based on a causal relationship (see sidebar). He wrote: "Here then are nine different viewpoints from all of which we should study association before we cry causation. What I do not believe—and this has been suggested—is that we can usefully lay down some hard and fast rules of evidence that must be obeyed before we can accept cause and effect." He noted that the mere postulate of confounders, unidentified, was not a valid reason to discount causality. He also stressed that a public policy decision on a hazard might have to be made before the evidence of a causal relationship was complete.

The criteria he suggested have recently been discussed in some detail by many authors. In 1988, a collection of essays on this question entitled *Causal Inference* was edited by Kenneth Rothman (84), and this book should be consulted by anyone interested in this important question. The discussion of each of Hill's criteria by Douglas Weed, Stephen Lanes, and others in Rothman's volume is too detailed for my present purposes. However, some observations will clarify the process in relation to the hazards we are considering.

In terms of the strength of an association, it is true that the stronger it is, the better evidence it provides toward causality. However, such factors as poor exposure measurement (as in the case of EMF), variability in outcome (such as in IQ determinations in children), or the fact that we are studying multifactorial disease (such as asthma), all will act to weaken what might otherwise be a strong association. In other words, unless exposure and outcome are well characterized, we cannot dismiss a "weak" association as necessarily representing reality. Indeed, Lanes (84) has argued that "the strength-of-association criterion, like other causal criteria, is an untestable tautology."

The criterion of temporality requires that the exposure precede the outcome. In arguing against a causal inference in relation to cigarettes and lung cancer, Sir Ronald Fisher suggested that the lung irritation caused by the cancer induced the desire to smoke, and hence that the cancer preceded the smoking (30).

In air pollution epidemiology, consistency is an important criterion. If particulate levels in time-series analyses are related to daily mortality in Chicago for example, the same should be true in Detroit, or Philadelphia, or wherever else the type of pollution is similar.

I have recently argued that coherence within different indices of adverse air pollution effects should be an important criterion of causal-

Criteria for a Causal Inference (from reference 85)

STRENGTH OF ASSOCIATION

CONSISTENCY: Observed by different people, in different places, circumstances, and times

SPECIFICITY: As in occupational exposures

TEMPORALITY: Exposure predates the outcome

BIOLOGIC GRADIENT: Dose-response curve

BIOLOGICAL PLAUSIBILITY: "This is a feature I am convinced we cannot demand" (Bradford Hill)

COHERENCE: Histopathological evidence (from smokers)—consistent with biology of the disease

EXPERIMENT: Effect of preventive action

ANALOGY: Argument from known effects from another agent

ity (86). Thus, if a particular pollutant is shown to be related to mortality in a time-series analysis, it would follow that the same pollutant should be related to hospital admissions. This would necessarily be the case unless all the excess mortality occurred at home, or if no disease was caused that was not fatal, both unlikely circumstances. In the 1952 London episode, not only was mortality increased, but there was a major concomitant increase in the demand for hospital beds, and visits to a family practice in the London area for acute respiratory disease increased (11). This type of coherence between different indices of morbidity and mortality should play an important part in the assessment of the causal relationship that may underlie time-series associations.

Biologic gradient, or the demonstration of a dose-response effect, is important, and was clearly evident in relation to cigarette smoking and outcomes such as lung cancer and emphysema. In general, it should be possible to show that the higher the exposure, the greater is the risk. It also applies to the effects of raised blood lead levels.

Biological plausibility commonly causes difficulty in the interpretation of epidemiological evidence. Bradford Hill (85) wrote, "This is a feature I am convinced we cannot demand." Some observers have declined to entertain a causal hypothesis in the case of EMF, because there is no biologic plausibility. Others argue that our knowledge of the process of induction of cancer is not yet complete enough that we can discount the influence of modifications in body function induced by EMF, even though these do not in themselves cause cancer. In the case of air pollution, damage from ozone is inherently biologically very plausible (18) because it has been shown to be an irritant gas that produces inflammation in the lung at very low concentrations. However, we do not know the mechanism that might link low levels of sulfur dioxide to adverse health effects, nor do we understand how small particulate pollution may produce its biologic effects. It is the different emphasis placed on biological plausibility that underlies many of the differences in judgment in relation to these issues.

Lead, in my opinion, is a special case. Although in general it is accepted that lead is a neurotoxin, we cannot expect to understand the precise way in which it may affect children's behavior or the development of intelligence, because our basic understanding of the growth and development of the brain is still too primitive. In this instance, therefore, it is reasonable to argue that the lack of biologic plausibility—if by that we mean a full understanding of the basic mechanism—should not be used as an argument against the causality of the association.

It is undeniable that people differ in their readiness to assume a causal relationship from an association. In table 3.1 I have suggested some biases in this process. If self-knowledge is the beginning of wisdom, this table should be useful. The public is generally biased towards making a causal inference. This comes about, I think, because we always search for explanations of events that occur to us. Samuel Pepys in his diary attributed a heavy cold to the fact that he had washed his feet two weeks before. Such a human tendency can be taken to extremes by those members of the public who have a "conspiracy theory" handy for every event. The media reflect this tendency and amplify it. Being unaware of the problems inherent in arguing causality from associations—and having too little time or space for a measured discussion—the causality is assumed if anyone postulates it. In my experience, bureaucrats in the parliamentary systems of the United Kingdom and Canada are generally biased *against* making a causal inference; the slow acceptance of the need to remove lead from gasoline in both countries illustrated this. Their "cousins" in the United States are, in my experience, more likely to be biased the other way—at least this was the case in relation to EMF. I have noted that animal toxicologists, who are able to control all variables in their experiments, generally seem to be biased against making causal inferences unless the mechanisms are fully understood. They, and others, may also be influenced by the idea that, since good science is necessarily cautious, being more cautious represents better science. This kind of primitive thinking often passes as wisdom.

The phrase "type 1 error" is often used to describe the error of saying that an association is significant when it is not; a "type 2 error" is to fail to reject a false null hypothesis—that is, to deny it is significant when it really is. Both of these phrases, strictly defined, apply only to the assessment of the strength of associations, but they are often loosely applied to denote that a true causal relationship has been rejected (type 2 error), or that causality has been falsely concluded from an association (type 1 error).

The Problem of Multifactorial Disease

Synchronous with the wider dispersion of all the hazards under consideration was the growing realization that a great deal of disease was "multifactorial" in origin. The belief that a single disease necessarily had a single cause died slowly. In one sense, the Western world, having successfully combated diseases such as pneumococcal pneumonia, malaria, and tuberculosis, in which single dominant agents could be identified, was left with a large residuum of diseases that have many origins.

Thus, in the case of coronary artery disease, the leading cause of mortality in the Western world, it was recognized that genetic factors expressed as familial predispositions increased the risk; that premature death was related to body weight; that hypertension worsened the prognosis; that cigarette smoking increased the risk; that dietary fat intake, in some people at least, also increased the risk; and so forth. Lung cancer incidence is dominated by cigarette smoking, but it is now recognized that the risk of lung cancer in a smoker is increased by exposure to radon, to asbestos, to arsenic, and possibly to air pollution. Bronchial asthma certainly has a genetic basis in children, but it is now recognized that this chronic condition may be acquired in

Table 3.1. On Making a Causal Inference from Associations

Public at large	Biased in favor
Media	Biased in favor
Bureaucrats (Parliamentary)	Biased against
Bureaucrats (US)	Biased in favor
Affected industry	Biased against (vested interest)
Scientists (who have worked in the field in question)	May be biased either for or against
Scientists (who have not worked in the field)	Should be able to form independent judgment
Animal toxicologists	Biased against
Lawyers	Depends who the client is
Juries	Likely to give benefit of the doubt to any victim

later life as a result of occupational exposures to such agents as western red cedar dust or diisocyanate compounds, or as a consequence of respiratory infections. A worsening of status in this disease might occur through a number of different influences, of which air pollution is but one.

These diseases, and many others, represent a much more complex world than the public or the media currently understand. In relation to known multifactorial disease, there are a number of important constraints, as follows:

1. It is not possible to assign percentage proportional "responsibility" for different factors. This has been excellently illustrated by Saracci (87) in the case of cigarette smoking and asbestos exposure. Using table 3.2, which gives the proportional incidence of lung cancer in smokers and nonsmokers who have been exposed or not exposed to asbestos, Saracci noted that the excess rate in those exposed only to asbestos is 47.1, but it is 590.3, or 12.5 times greater, in the group exposed to both agents. He continued:

> Should the analysis stop here, the conclusion would almost automatically follow that in a situation as that por-

Table 3.2. Lung Cancer Risk with Smoking and Asbestos Exposure

Exposure Group	Death Rate (1)	Excess Rate (2)	% Excess Rate Removable by Eliminating	
			Smoking (3)	Asbestos (4)
A− S−	11.3	0.0	—	—
A+ S−	58.4	47.1	—	100.0
A− S+	122.6	111.3	100.0	—
A+ S+	601.6	590.3	92.0	81.2

From reference 87. See text for the correct interpretation of these data.

trayed by the death rates in column (1), smoking is by far the dominant factor, and its removal is, correspondingly, by far more effective as a preventive measure than asbestos removal. That things are not so simple is indicated by columns (3) and (4). If smoking is removed, the excess rate will go down from 590.3 to 47.1 i.e. some 543 lives will be saved (per 100,000 person years) or 92% of the excess rate will be removed. If, on the other hand, asbestos is removed, the excess rate will go down from 590.3 to 111.3, i.e., 479 lives will be saved, or 81.2% of the excess rate will be removed. This means that removal of smoking is more effective than removal of asbestos, but only 1.14 times (543/479) and not 12.5 times as it superficially appeared.

2. It follows from this that, when we know that a disease is multifactorial in origin, we should be very cautious of any statement telling us that 90 percent of the cases are caused by smoking. What might be the case is that 90 percent of the cases would not have occurred without smoking, but this does not mean that only 10 percent of cases are caused by something else. It might be that 85 percent of the cases would not have occurred if another agent had not been present, but people continued to smoke. One finds statements in the press or on television programs that do not recognize this basic limitation when a disease is known to be multifactorial. We are confidently told every day, "Obesity is responsible for 20 percent of all heart attacks"; or, "5 percent of all cancers are occupational in origin." Harrison and Hoberg (88) have recently documented this error in the case

of radon, noting that a Canadian Health and Welfare official "assumed that 90% of lung cancer deaths are caused by smoking, and that 5% of lung cancer deaths occur 'spontaneously,' leaving a residual of up to 5% which could possibly be ascribed to radon exposure."

3. Checkoway and Hickey (89) have presented an elegant statistical and algebraic analysis of this problem in multifactorial disease. Their paper should be required reading by students in environmental health sciences.

4. There is no doubt that this problem leads to serious difficulties in disease attribution. All those who have developed risk estimates of cancer from asbestos exposure agree that the number of lung cancers induced will be at least twice as many as cases of mesothelioma. In British Columbia, in the years 1980 to 1988 inclusive, the Workers' Compensation Board recognized sixty-nine cases of mesothelioma. During the same period, only eleven cases of lung cancer were recognized in which asbestos exposure was considered to have contributed to the risk. This disparity was not because cases were rejected by the board, but because cases of lung cancer were never brought forward, since the doctors presumably thought that smoking alone had caused the disease. The question of whether the patient would have developed lung cancer without asbestos exposure was presumably never asked. It was calculated in 1986 that approximately two thousand mesothelioma and between four thousand and six thousand lung cancer deaths that would not have occurred without asbestos exposure were occurring annually in the United States (90).

5. In both the United States and Canada, mortality from heart disease has fallen over the past eight years. Do we know how much of this change is to be attributed to reduced smoking, or to jogging, or to less fat in the diet, or to better immediate care? All we know is that we cannot ascribe the effects in percentages so that they will add up to 100 percent. For similar reasons, we cannot apportion the factors responsible for asthma in order to make statements like, "5 percent of asthma is due to air pollution." This principle operates in other fields. In a recent article (91), Stephen Jay Gould wrote the following note in an article on evolution:

> Incidentally, the concept of emergence helps us to understand why the nature-nurture issue is such a false dichotomy. Genes influence many aspects of human behavior,

but we cannot say that such behavior is caused by genes in any direct way. We cannot even claim that a given behavior is, say, 40 percent genetic and 60 percent environmental, and thereby defend at least a partial old-fashioned genetic determinism. Genes and environment interact in a nonadditive way, yielding emergent features in the resulting anatomies, physiologies, and behaviors.

6. Rose (92) has pointed out that, if we imagine a country in which everyone smoked ten cigarettes a day, we would conclude that lung cancer had a genetic basis. In a sense this would be true, since with everyone smoking but only some getting lung cancer, some factors must determine which members of the population get the disease and which do not. The more widely distributed a factor is, the more difficult it is to determine its role in any multifactorial disease in which we know it exerts an influence. In Chapter 2, the question was asked, "How we can determine the present role of environmental asbestos exposure in relation to lung cancer, when the lungs of city dwellers not occupationally exposed to the material are found to contain millions of asbestos fibers?" With 86 million Americans currently exposed to levels of ozone higher than the EPA standard, how are we to determine whether this is influencing the prevalence or severity of asthma? These are complex questions because of the difficulty of describing multifactorial disease.

7. Understanding the problem of multifactorial causation is very important when media reporters, with their short attention span and thirst for the dramatic statement, try to badger anyone not on his or her guard into saying, "50 percent of all cases of asthma are due to . . ."

8. Another issue is the common, but almost certainly false, assumption that diseases we do not currently understand are not multifactorial in origin. Have we any reason to assume that childhood leukemia has one cause? Theriault (75) noted the possibility that EMF was one of a number of factors that increased the risk of cancer. Possibly it is the combination of EMF exposure and concomitant exposure to hydrocarbons from automobile or diesel exhaust. If so, these factors might not be "confounders" in the ordinary sense, but additional factors contributing to the risk.

Once the reality of multifactorial disease is grasped, many oversimplified statements (even some made by distinguished people) can be

identified as essentially misleading. There is no doubt that a sophisticated approach to multifactorial disease is required when most issues
in environmental health are being considered.

The Role of Risk Assessment and Perception

The past twenty years have seen a major expansion in formal risk
assessment activity. Corn (93) has recently written an excellent review
of the developing role of risk assessment in relation to occupational
hazards between 1970 and 1990. A complete review of this discipline
would not be germane to my present purpose. However, the process
of risk assessment has become so central to any consideration of public hazards, and is so likely to affect future policy decisions, that some
description of it is obligatory. The following points will serve as an
introduction.

   1. It is not possible to conduct a formal risk assessment unless there
is some capability of constructing a dose-response relationship. The calculations of public risk from environmental asbestos exposure shown
in table 2.7 depend on downward extrapolation from occupational exposure data. Risk calculations in the absence of such information (as is
the present case in relation to EMF) can only be expressed as risk ratios.

   2. As shown in table 2.8, there may be a considerable range of risk
estimates. In such instances, a mean value may be taken as broadly
representative of the whole. Rosenthal, Gray, and Graham (94) have
recently published a detailed and scholarly review of the process of
risk assessment as applied to carcinogenic chemicals. They wrote:

> In summary, in spite of its appearance of precision, QRA
> (quantitative risk assessment) is fraught with gaps in
> knowledge that are filled with guesses and assumptions.
> Risk assessors have a great deal of analytical discretion in
> the conduct of cancer risk assessments. As we have dis-
> cussed, the choice and interpretation of data, the choice of
> extrapolation models, and the choice of exposure assump-
> tions and models can make a huge difference in the out-
> come of a risk assessment. . . .
>
>   Regardless of one's theory of democracy, our analysis of
> the risk assessment process suggests that mandated risk
> levels per se would do little to assert democratic control

over the standard setting process. The numerous semi-technical, semipolicy judgements pervasive in the calculation of carcinogenic risk could frustrate any congressional attempt to control regulatory decisions through specification of risk levels.

We saw, for example, that alternative choices of exposure assumptions and dose-response models can lead to plausible risk estimates that vary by several orders of magnitude. If agency officials believe that a statutory bright line is too stringent in a particular case, they can manipulate the risk calculation to produce a numerical estimate of risk that will allow them to justify their desired level of stringency.

3. Table 3.3 shows the odds ratios for two different levels of cumulative exposure to coal dust in a large cohort of United States coal miners (95). It can be seen that, in relation to symptom prevalence and lung function, increased cumulative exposure leads to a greater risk of depressed lung function and of various symptoms. When large data banks exist that can be analyzed in this way, a convincing estimate of risk relation to exposure can be displayed. Such estimates, based on reliable exposure and outcome data, do not suffer from the difficulties in risk estimation noted in the paragraph above.

4. Major difficulties in risk estimation occur when animal toxicological data (often concerning induced cancers) are to be converted to a human risk estimate. In view of known species differences, it is to be expected that these limitations will continue.

5. Long latency periods, such as that existing in the case of mesothelioma following asbestos exposure, present difficulties, as the period of observation may be too short for all the induced cases to be detected. For example, a recent report from Göteborg (96), in a prospective study of shipyard workers seven to fifteen years after all exposure to asbestos had ceased, found that mesotheliomas were still occurring at approximately ten times the expected rate.

The development of risk estimates has been paralleled by interest in the public perception of risk and what influences it, and more recently in "risk communication." Upton (97) has recently summarized much of this material, and table 3.4 is taken from his recent discussion. The differentiation between characteristics that seem to

Table 3.3. Odds Ratios for Exposure to 1 and 20 mg/m^3-Years
Coal Mine Dust Based on Logistic Regression Models

	OR$_1$[a] (95% C.I.)[a]	OR$_{20}$[a]
FEV$_1$ <80%	1.03 (1.01,1.06)	1.9
FEV$_1$/FVC <80%	1.05 (1.01,1.09)	2.5
Cough	1.02 (0.99,1.04)	1.4
Phlegm	1.03 (1.01,1.05)	1.8
Chronic bronchitis	1.02 (1.00,1.05)	1.6
Obstructive bronchitis	1.04 (1.00,1.08)	2.0
Breathlessness	1.03 (1.01,1.05)	1.8
Wheeze	1.03 (1.01,1.05)	1.7
Wheeze with SOB	1.03 (1.01,1.06)	1.9

[a]Odds ratio as determined by the logistic models given in Table III for the increase in exposure of 1, and 20 mg/m^3-years.

From reference 95. Note the progressively higher risks of respiratory symptoms or a lowered FEV1 with a twenty-fold increase in cumulative coal dust exposure. Where exposure data is reasonably precise, such calculations provide an excellent guide to the maximal exposure that should be permitted.

increase the public acceptability of a risk, such as when it is voluntarily undertaken, or familiar, and characteristics that tend to decrease the acceptability of risk, such as when it is presented by an untrusted source or is undetectable by the individual, provide a useful summary of much previous investigation. Such characteristics strike a chord in most thinking people.

What is often not emphasized is that all of us are used to making personal decisions that are based on our perception of risk, but are uninfluenced by statistical considerations. I may decide, at the age of sixty, that it is no longer "safe" for me to use a chain saw when up a tree. I base this on my perceptions of my own strength and reaction time; I may make such a reasonable judgment in the absence of any knowledge of the statistics of injuries to people more than sixty years old under these conditions. In a perhaps more familiar example, we may go out to dinner in the winter and visit a couple who live ten miles up a remote and difficult road. While we are having dinner, it begins to snow hard, and when it is time to leave, six inches have fallen. Our host suggests that we stay the night, and return in the morning. An immediate "yes" or "no" decision has to be made. In milliseconds, we assess the state of our tires, our knowledge of the road, our commitments early tomorrow, and even our estimate of the state of our blood alcohol, and either accept his invitation or decide to make the journey.

Table 3.4. Psychosocial and Cultural Characteristics Affecting the Perception of Risk

Characteristics That Tend to Increase Acceptability of a Risk	Characteristics That Tend to Decrease Acceptability of a Risk
Voluntary	Involuntary
Familiar	Unfamiliar
Immediate impact	Remote impact
Detectable by individual	Nondetectable by individual
Controllable by individual	Uncontrollable by individual
Fair	Unfair
Noncatastrophic	Catastrophic
Well understood	Poorly understood
Natural	Artificial
Trusted source	Untrusted source
Visible benefits	No visible benefits

Source: Slovic et al. (1979); Plough and Krimsky (1987).

From reference (97). Although based on a considerable volume of carefully collected data, these categories generally correspond with our intuitive feelings.

We are therefore used to having to make personal choices based on the best information available to us, but uninformed by statistical data. What purpose do the statistical estimates of risk shown in table 2.8 serve? The answer is that they provide a necessary basis for public policy decisions, such as whether and if asbestos should be removed; whether present coal dust standards are adequately protective; whether automobile lead represents an unacceptable hazard; and so on. There can be no doubt that such estimates are essential prior to policy determination, but they have always to be interpreted with knowledge of their limitations.

In instances in which the public expresses a greater fear than is justified on the basis of comparative risk estimates (as in the case of nuclear power, for example), can it be assumed that all that is required is more education, and people will then change their opinion on policy? On the basis of the public response to the Chernobyl disaster, this seems to me very unlikely. Indeed, when that event occurred, many members of the public took the view that this catastrophic event confirmed their "hunch"—as against the formal risk estimates of the experts—that the technology was too potentially dangerous to be widely deployed. In this case, therefore, risk communication is very likely to be viewed by some members of the public as biased "education" by a highly partisan group of interests, and this is unquestionably what it can become. At its best however, risk communication can be a consensus-building and consultative exercise, and can play an important part in decision making as a result.

There is no doubt that objectivity, as represented by formal risk assessment, will remain an important component of decision making. Where an environmental impact assessment is to be conducted (on hazards from a new incinerator for example), certain prior conditions should be met. The first is that the objective risk assessment should be prepared by individuals who have no financial stake in the project; the second is that this risk assessment should be critiqued in public by a second independent group; and the third is that this process should be in the public domain, with those members of the public who are likely to be impacted able to ask questions of both the proposer and the risk assessors.

Economic Aspects of Environmental Policy Decisions

A few weeks after the London air pollution episode in December 1952, the government expressed concern that it would be far too expensive to take the steps that might be required to prevent a repetition of the incident. However, in spite of this, for the next fifteen years or so, it was common to hear the attitude expressed that, if public damage could be shown to be occurring, then it was incumbent upon government to take the requisite action to put a stop to it. I can recall assuming that this would necessarily be the position of every right-minded citizen.

It later became popular to argue that, before any preventive action should be taken, it had to be proved that the benefit from the proposed action outweighed the costs of taking it. However, a special report to Congress in 1989 (98) examined the health benefits from the reduction of air pollution and wrote: "We conclude that though there is no doubt that significant health benefits result from controlling some air pollutants, it is not currently feasible to produce an unambiguous evaluation of the health benefits."

Nevertheless, detailed attempts have been made to compute some benefits of reducing air pollution. Thus, the United States Environmental Protection Agency argued that the reduction in male blood pressure that would follow the removal of lead from gasoline more than compensated for the costs of taking the action. They did not place a specific dollar amount on a unit of IQ in a child (which, in my opinion, would hardly have been ethically possible), but they did calculate the costs of the supplemental education required for impaired children. In 1985, the EPA issued a paper on the health benefits calculable from removing lead from gasoline (99). For the year 1988, it was computed that, from the point of view of children's health, the benefits would be $502 million; by reduction of blood pressure in adults, the benefits would total $5 billion; and the total monetized benefits amounted to $6.2 billion. By contrast, the costs to the refining industry were calculated to be only $532 million. Thus, the EPA argued that the economic benefit of the reduction in male blood pressure that would follow the removal of lead from gasoline more than compensated for the costs of taking the action.

In relation to photochemical air pollution, Hall and her colleagues in Los Angeles (100) have recently published a very detailed estimate of health costs attributable to air pollution in that city. This required placing dollar costs on symptoms such as cough and chest tightness consequent upon photochemical air pollution. Even without taking any account of possible long-term effects, they computed the health benefits of attaining the United States ozone standard as between $1.2 and $5.8 billion annually, with a best estimate of $2.7 billion. For the particulate PM10 (fine particles less than 10 microns in size) standard, since they computed mortality costs in relation to this, the best estimate total was $6.4 billion. Another economist has recently argued that ozone controls are currently too expensive for the United States to contemplate (101).

Such exercises have the merit of indicating the extent of air pollution problems by putting a dollar figure on public discomfort or actual morbidity. In the case of asbestos, no attempt has been made to put a dollar figure on the health effects of environmental asbestos. This would require some basic assumptions, such as attributing all of the 30 percent of mesothelioma cases without prior occupational exposure to environmental asbestos inhalation, and this would immediately be challenged. On the basis of our present knowledge, the matter could evidently not be settled.

The report to Congress quoted above (98) indicated that there was a third perspective on economic costs in relation to pollution. In this, benefits in terms of health effects avoided are compared, so that the best decisions can be taken about which pollutants require most emphasis.

It is not clear whether strict economic analyses can, or for that matter should, provide the basis for environmental decision making. I have always thought that, once it has been agreed that raised blood lead levels in children impair intellectual development, and that there is no demonstrable threshold, it is mandatory that the exposure of children to lead should be reduced as much as possible. I find it immoral to try to put a dollar cost on the disbenefit of a lowered IQ in a child. The only question, therefore, is whether the association demonstrated between mental effects and blood lead represents a causal relationship; once that judgment has been made, the need for the removal of lead from gasoline should not have to be argued on other grounds. For this reason, in 1972, I wrote that, on the basis of the evidence then, lead had to be removed from gasoline (7).

Events in eastern Europe have shown that it is possible at the same time to have both a grossly degraded environment and economic collapse. It used to be argued that the choice was always between pollution control and "jobs," representing a flourishing economy. M.E. Porter of the Harvard University Business School has recently called this philosophy into question by pointing to examples in which the countries with the tightest pollution controls have the most efficient industries (102). This may come about because an industry may be forced to modernize to meet new pollution standards, and in the process may develop a far more efficient manufacturing plant. Curtis Moore (103) has also criticized the "jobs versus the environment" argument, still believed by many in the business community.

These arguments will no doubt continue to evolve in free societies. They will remain important in relation to policy, but the attitudes taken may well differ between countries, and within individual countries, with different government leadership at different times.

The 1990 amendments to the Clean Air Act of 1970 in the United States are 328 pages long, and their detail and complexity are far greater than in any previous legislation. Curtis Moore, in an exhaustive analysis of the amendments, has recently written (104):

> Tension between protection of the environment and public health on the one hand and considerations of cost and convenience on the other are common in environmental

decision making. The 1970 Clean Air Act Amendments resolved that tension in favor of protection of health and the
environment, forcing changes in technology and behavior
where necessary. The principal author of the 1970 amendments, Sen. Edward S. Muskie, said as the Senate began
consideration of the proposals:

"The first responsibility of Congress is not the making of
technological or economic judgments—or even to be limited by what is or appears to be technologically or economically feasible. Our responsibility is to establish what the
public interest requires to protect the health of persons.
This may mean that people and industries will be asked to
do what seems to be impossible at the present time. But if
health is to be protected, these challenges must be met. I
am convinced they can be met."

In contrast, the 1990 amendments resolve that tension
between protection and costs and convenience in favor of
the latter, with the result that alleged limits of technology
constrain the level of protection. Thus the law as altered by
the 1990 amendments is a significantly different creature
from the 1970 Act. After amendment, protection of human
health has all but ceased to be the basis of the law. . . .

If this reading of the 1990 amendments is correct, it signals an
important (but little noted) change of principle behind environmental
legislation in the United States. That this reflects the attitude of the
current (1992) administration is supported by other recent actions,
such as the refusal of the EPA to review the ozone standard, and the
government's refusal to sign certain international agreements at the
recent United Nations conference in Rio de Janeiro.

4

A Survival Kit for the Environmental Jungle

Following the examination of the five hazards, and the description of some special problems associated with environmental health risks, special attention can now be directed to the main players. These are individual scientists, legislators, lawyers, industry, media, and the public. It is clear that one of the main problems of public health protection is in the accurate description of epidemiological data; since this involves all the players, it will be discussed first.

Interpreting Epidemiological Data

Before a body of epidemiological data can be expressed in a general summary, words have to be chosen to describe as exactly as possible what the speaker judges to be the strength or weakness of the data. In the sidebar, six different phrases are used to describe epidemiological results. The first, that the data "unanimously indicate a highly significant association" might apply to a review of studies of cigarette smoking and lung cancer. It indicates that all studies show a strong association. The second statement, "generally indicate a significant association," would be suitable for certain air pollution and general morbidity studies; it might also be used for the studies of association between blood lead and neurobehavioral changes in children. The last four statements (see box) are taken from different comments on the health data relating to EMF, and suggest greater or lesser degrees of skepticism.

Such statements deal only with the degree of confidence that the

---

Interpreting Epidemiological Data

Comparative strength of the words used:
The epidemiological data we have reviewed—
- "unanimously indicate a highly significant association"
- "generally indicate a significant association"
- "indicate a weak association between . . ."
- "tend to suggest an association"
- "while indicating a possible association, have demonstrated only a weak relationship"
- "results . . . appear to provide some weak evidence in support of the postulated association"

The first of these might apply to the relationship between cigarette smoking and lung cancer. The last three are all taken from recent reports on the possible carcinogenicity of electromagnetic fields.

---

speaker (or committee) may have in relation to the association. It is important that any comment on policy or its implications be separated from the statement on the force or weakness of the data. The following sentence was quoted in Chapter 2 from the British Medical Research Council Advisory Committee report on lead (50):

> While the observed statistical associations detailed in this review are consistent with the hypothesis that low-level lead exposure has a small negative effect on the performance of children in ability and attainment tests, the limitations of epidemiological studies in drawing causal inferences are such that it is not possible to conclude that exposure to lead at current urban levels is definitely harmful.

Such a paragraph requires detailed analysis. The first sentence concedes that associations of lead and lowered IQ and performance have been shown to occur, but by using the word "small" encourages the view that it can be neglected. The second sentence suggests that these results can be ignored on account of "the limitations of epidemiological studies." One wonders which aspect of Hill's suggested causal criteria is being referred to here. The end of the paragraph might mean either that blood lead levels in children are not adversely affected by the lead in automobile exhaust or that the studies show effects only at levels above those that might be acquired in urban living (i.e., that a threshold has been found). It is obvious that, without much more detailed discussion, the suggested conclusion about urban lead levels cannot be assumed to follow the earlier conclusion drawn from the epidemiological studies that were reviewed. If the paragraph was intended simply to reassure the inexpert reader, it might succeed in its purpose. As a precise statement of the current issues raised by lead exposure, it leaves a lot to be desired.

This example indicates the importance of very precise and exact wording when describing the results of epidemiological studies and the conclusions the writer is drawing from them. If it is suggested that a conclusion has been reached as a result of reviewing such studies, which has certain policy implications, these studies should be discussed separately. Furthermore, as I have noted earlier, the set of values behind the final opinion must be explicitly articulated. The reader should not be left to guess why he or she might come to a different conclusion.

In table 3.1, I suggested that certain biases existed in relation to the interpretation of epidemiological data. One can make a case for concluding that special committees in the United Kingdom, and possibly also in Canada, are less likely to conclude that an association is causal than are their counterparts in the United States. But if a committee anywhere is large enough, on any controversial issue its members are very likely to differ in opinion on the question of causation. Furthermore, the larger the representation of "basic" scientists, the greater the tendency to dismiss associative data (this follows from table 3.2). This is largely because scientific methodology, as in animal toxicology studies, is designed to eliminate variables and produce direct evidence of causation. Finding words to accommodate a range of opinion within such a committee can be time consuming and difficult. Yet the task is unquestionably important.

Mistakes Made by Scientists

Leaving aside all cases in which scientists are paid to express opinions favorable to one view of epidemiological data, one can identify four classes of mistakes commonly made (see sidebar). The last of these, "failure to recognize that emotion is an appropriate force for policy change," is very common. On an occasion many years ago, when I was arguing for a policy based only on reason, Bruce Doern, then director of the School of Public Administration at Carleton University, pointed out to me that emotion was a proper force in relation to policy, and this is unquestionably correct, though easy to forget in the world of experimental data and risk analysis.

Salter (58), in discussing the process of inquiry into the toxicity of the pesticide Captan, refers to evidence given by scientists and conclusions reached. She writes:

> The second statement, "We have no evidence that the pesticide captan is dangerous to human populations," is not hypothetical, but is taken from the discussions about the final report of the expert committee on captan. In the scientific discourse about captan, this statement is not very interesting and in the context of the expert committee report, this statement was accurate. Since only toxicological data existed about captan at the time this statement was made, and since toxicological experiments used animal populations, there could have been no scientific evidence that captan was actually dangerous to humans. All that was available to the expert committee were extrapolations from animal studies by scientists who differed in their interpretation of the data."

As noted in Chapter 2, most scientists are now sensitive to the fine line between an estimate of the force of scientific data on the one hand, and an opinion based on a value judgment on the other. It is important that, whenever public statements are being made, the language accurately reflects this sensitivity. As I have pointed out elsewhere (105), it is common that a defensible difference in opinion between scientists—as to how certain data are to be interpreted—is wrongly portrayed by the media as evidence that the process of scientific inquiry is thereby discredited.

It is also important to distinguish between concluding that a stage has been reached when steps should be taken to reduce the levels of lead exposure in a community, and telling individual parents that their child has been adversely affected by lead. This latter situation is what the television crew would like, as the family can then be inter-

---

Mistakes Made by Scientists

Mistaken judgment on probability of causation

Mistaken assessment of reliability of the data (Note bias against credibility of epidemiological data in most experimental scientists)

Failure to distinguish between scientific knowledge and policy judgment

Failure to recognize that emotion is an appropriate force for policy change

Examples of all of these are noted in the text.

---

viewed and the whole complex problem reduced to "one-on-one" terms. It is perfectly proper to say publicly that such a stage has been reached in terms of the community, but to refuse to identify individual cases that may have been affected by the risk. Environmental scientists must clearly understand this differentiation.

Role of the Media

As indicated in table 2.1, in a free society the media play a dominant role in public education on environmental questions. Historically, they have been important in drawing attention to actual and potential environmental health problems. Unexplained clusters of disease, apparent increases in disease prevalence, summarizing official reports or legal cases involving cigarette smoking or asbestos exposure—in all these instances the media are responsible for informing the public and alerting the legislator. It is clear that anyone involved in trying to understand environmental health issues cannot avoid the responsibility of responding to requests from the media for information or explanation. However, the four negative points shown in the sidebar must be fully understood by anyone who collaborates with the media. I have rarely said anything publicly about an environmental issue without the first question from reporters being: "Is air pollution a more important problem than . . . ?" Arranging all problems in some order of priority seems to be a preoccupation of some interviewers. Such questions should never be answered. If you are an asthmatic living in a modern city, air pollution may be more important to you than the

Role of the Media

Dominant role in relation to public perceptions: (Incoming medical students identify the media as the main source of their information on environmental health)

Generally reflect and amplify all signals

Always oversimplify complex issues

Often stress false "priority" criteria

These factors, especially the last three, must be well understood (and expected) by scientists who try to provide balanced input to the media.

effect of lead on the intelligence of children; if you live close to a lead smelter, questions of the effect of EMF might well be secondary. There is, therefore, no generic order of priority applicable to everyone to which all questions conform.

Media personnel have great difficulty in understanding the limitations imposed on anyone who discusses multifactorial disease. Also, they do not appreciate that answering the question "How many people in Vancouver take *The New Yorker?*" is different from the answer to "How many people in Vancouver are affected by air pollution?" Also, in their minds all percentages have to add up to a hundred, which, as noted earlier, is not true of potential causative factors in multifactorial disease. Nevertheless, it is the important and essential task of the media in a free society to assist the public, and through them the legislators, to determine that the weight of evidence has shifted the burden of proof in relation to a specific question, such as that of the relationship between cigarettes and lung cancer.

Role of the Corporate Lawyer

The lawyer commissioned to make the strongest case on behalf of his or her client cannot be expected to emphasize aspects of the evidence that point in a different direction. In the sidebar I have listed four aspects of a legal defense that should be anticipated. Attempts have been made (most notably by Milton Wessel [106]) to suggest that, in some circumstances, ethical considerations should override these attitudes, but

---

Influence of the Corporate Lawyer

Deny any responsibility

Point out that the epidemiological data do not constitute proof

Argue that confounders have influenced the epidemiological association

Suggest the presence of unidentified confounders

Argue that there is no biological plausibility for the alleged effect

Note: Will often use any method (short of force) to discredit the evidence of opposing expert witnesses

Reference 106 should be consulted for a scholarly discussion of some of these factors. These points are based on my own experience, however.

---

there is little evidence that this advice has been heeded. The scientist who strays into this minefield must be aware that attempts to throw doubt on his or her credibility are to be expected. It is apparently inherent in all legal training that any points you can score against the character of the witness should be scored, even if these have nothing to do with the question in hand. More subtle is the attempt to get an expert scientific witness to go beyond the strict questions on which he or she is expert, or to get him or her to represent as a "fact" something that is really only an opinion. When the financial stakes are enormous, as is the case with asbestos, all of these devices will be used without scruple. The relationship between "science" and the "legal process" has been viewed as a shotgun marriage, and there is no doubt that there are aspects of each that contravene the standards of the other. The environmental scientist requires considerable judgment in how answers are phrased. It is all too easy to be pushed into a statement that is too dogmatic for the weight of evidence, or to be so cautious that a judge is entitled to the conclusion that the court is unlikely to learn anything of value from the witness.

The role of industrial consortia (no doubt guided by their corporate lawyers) has varied in relation to these five hazards. The tobacco industry has fought efforts to limit or reduce cigarette smoking in every free society, and has no conscience about promoting cigarette consumption in the Third World. The asbestos industry's attitude to

Because it Counts

its unquestionable responsibility is a matter of record (45). The removal of lead from gasoline was, quite understandably, strongly opposed by the industry that made tetraethyl lead. Interested industries have generally opposed stricter air pollution legislation. In the case of electromagnetic fields, the industry has not engaged in "dirty tricks" or in efforts to discredit epidemiologists. If stronger epidemiological data are published, or if restrictive legislation is proposed, this attitude might be expected to change.

Societies supported by the public stand on the other side of the argument. They are subject to the temptation to exaggerate the data, as this is required if fund raising from a concerned public is to continue. The scientist or physician who attempts some kind of balance or objectivity in relation to these questions often finds him- or herself in a "no-man's land" between these opposing forces, cowering in a shell hole while the missiles pass overhead.

Phrases to Watch Out for

The four phrases listed in the sidebar occur repeatedly in hearings, debates, and press releases on all environmental hazards in which the data are either incomplete or contradictory.

If a counsel states, "There is no scientific proof that . . . ," he or she should be immediately asked what, in his or her opinion, would constitute scientific proof that the effect existed. Is a scientific consensus meant? Is "proof" used in a mathematical sense? What proof commonly exists for any biological phenomena? Does he or she consider that it has been proven that cigarettes cause lung cancer?

Much the same line of questioning should follow a statement that "there is no statistical proof that . . ."

The phrase "No significant excess of . . ." is commonly used to describe an increase in an observed incidence over what would be expected, when this finding is inconvenient to the speaker. The incidence often requires much more careful definition than the speaker gives. If the increased cases are considered to represent a random cluster, then this should be precisely stated. If other clusters seem to be occurring elsewhere in relation to the same exposure, more explanation is required. It is easy to dismiss one cluster as representing "no significant excess of . . . ," but harder to explain the occurrence of similar clusters wherever the hazard can be identified.

Phrases to Watch Out for

"No scientific proof that . . ."

"No statistical proof that . . ."

"No significant excess of . . ."

"No objective evidence of . . ."

> Whenever any of these phrases is used in a discussion of epidemiological data, as noted in the text, some additional questions must immediately be put to the speaker.

Public Health Decision Making in a Free Society

The example of the very serious adverse health effects of cigarette smoking suggests that the process of public decision making in a free society follows the following sequence of events:

Stage 1. Initial epidemiological evidence begins to suggest a strong association between cigarettes and lung cancer. No one study constitutes "proof." Prospective studies may be stronger than retrospective ones.

Stage 2. A stage is reached when epidemiological studies in different countries, conducted in different ways, all show a strong association. It becomes difficult to think of a common confounder. As Bradford Hill (85) remarked in this context:

> But to explain the pronounced excess in cancer of the lung in any other environmental terms requires some feature of life so intimately linked with cigarette smoking and with the amount of smoking that such a feature should be easily detectable. If we cannot detect it or reasonably infer a specific one, then in such circumstances I think we are reasonably entitled to reject the vague contention of the armchair critic, "you can't prove it, there may be such a feature." . . .
>
> What I do not believe—and this has been suggested—is that we can usefully lay down some hard-and-fast rules of evidence that must be obeyed before we accept cause and

effect. None of my nine viewpoints can bring indisputable evidence for or against the cause-and-effect hypothesis and none can be required as a sine qua non. What they can do, with greater or less strength, is to help us make up our minds on the fundamental question—is there any other way of explaining the set of facts before us, is there any other answer equally, or more, likely than cause and effect?

Stage 3. When the body of data is large enough, the burden of proof shifts from those who have to prove causality to those (from the tobacco industry, in the case of cigarettes) who argue that the epidemiological data do not permit a judgment of causality. Such proponents should be required to offer an explanation of why so much epidemiological evidence points in the same direction. This process can be facilitated by a carefully structured public inquiry at which questions of this kind can be put. As noted earlier in this chapter, the role of the media is essential in establishing that this point has been reached.

Stage 4. When this stage is reached (perhaps in 1963 in the case of cigarettes), government or regulatory intervention is required.

The media are so central in these questions because it is only through media presentations and discussion that a free society can finally reach an "opinion" that causality is no longer in doubt. Until this stage is reached, public opinion is unlikely to support action to curb the risk (smoking level, in this case).

This scenario seems to have been relevant to cigarette smoking, but it is not at all clear that it applies universally. Indeed, Rose (92) has pointed out that the example of cigarettes, with its exceptionally strong epidemiological background, may have misled us as to the way in which we have to regard other environmental hazards. In the case of air pollution, the dialogue does occur in the media episodically, particularly in the worst affected regions, but the attainment of anything approaching a national consensus would seem unlikely. In the case of lead, government action was taken after representations by scientists that attracted very little media or public attention.

The question of the hazard of environmental asbestos has been almost entirely taken over by the courts. Discussion of the validity of risk estimates, and of dust levels within buildings, occurs mainly in relation to specific litigation. This phenomenon has made scientific dialogue in the public arena, between those who hold opposite points of view, almost impossible. The Health Effects Institute report (47) was mandated by the U.S. Congress in an effort to provide a relatively objective review of contemporary data. In the case of electromagnetic fields, it has been possible to argue that the data do not yet provide a sufficiently strong foundation for legislative or other action, though this might change as a result of the new studies from Sweden (78, 79).

Summary

The sidebar summarizes the mistakes and misunderstandings that can be easily identified from the five environmental hazards. A full understanding of them and familiarity with them is, I believe, an essential requirement in the equipment any environmental health professional must have for survival in the environmental jungle.

Mistakes and Misunderstandings

1. Misunderstanding the interface between "science" and "values."
2. Underrating the importance to public health of "small" changes in mean values when the population exposed is large.
3. Denying a causal relationship in presence of significant associations.
4. Not understanding the constraints on making a causal inference from associations.
5. Not understanding that poor exposure data and other factors may weaken an association.
6. Misunderstanding the nature of scientific "proof."
7. Not understanding the complexity of multifactorial disease.

5

Conclusions

A contemporary visitor to the Western industrial democracies from the Third World or from eastern Europe might well conclude that the democratic process has shown itself over the past forty years to be capable of containing many risks to public health. As a result of government initiative, publicity, and restrictions on advertising, general cigarette consumption has fallen. Air pollution from coal burning has been greatly reduced, and although automobile-generated pollution has yet to be controlled, it has not been shown to have severe and direct effects on health, though the ozone generated from these emissions probably is a hazard. Indeed, reviewing air pollution, both Dr. Merrill Eisenbud (107) in the United States and Sir Richard Doll (38) in Britain have concluded that serious adverse health effects are no longer being caused by air pollution. Legislation has forbidden the use of asbestos in buildings, and its handling and removal is subject to strict supervision. The general use of asbestos has declined dramatically. Lead has been removed from gasoline, and is no longer a serious air pollutant in the Western world. Exposure to electromagnetic fields has not yet been conclusively shown to be an important factor in disease (though the accumulation of such evidence is disquieting).

The visitor might therefore review all these potential health risks and conclude that the democratic process has shown itself sensitive and responsive to each of these issues as they have arisen.

There is, however, another side to this issue. There is a difference between dramatic events, like the excess mortality in the 1952 episode in London, and the aggravation of a common condition such as asthma. Also, it is still too early to expect that the full consequences of oxidant air pollution, when a huge population is exposed, should be understood. Cigarette smoking is still common in some young people, especially in young women, in some countries. Asbestos exposure, as judged by the load of asbestos in the lungs of city dwellers, is still occurring; and the consequences of this are still controversial. It is still too early to know that legislative action is required to limit exposure to electromagnetic fields. The removal of lead from gasoline stands out, perhaps, as an unqualified success, but in this case it is unclear how powerful an influence the health risks were in that decision.

It would be difficult, however, to convince a perceptive visitor that the process of decision making had been orderly, rational, and consecutive. Much seems to have depended either on unpredictable and episodic media interest, or on dedicated efforts by individual scientists and legislators. Yet, on reflection, perhaps one should expect that in a democracy, however flawed, much of the decision making would necessarily be haphazard and appear to be disorganized. In the protection of public health from these hazards, it is the freedom of expression within the society, together with access to information, that is crucial.

We can distinguish four distinct stages in relation to these five hazards:

Stage 1. First epidemiological study; disbelief.

Stage 2. More epidemiological data confirm original study; search for biological mechanisms begins. "Causality not proven until mechanism is understood."

Stage 3. Significant association confirmed in all studies, burden of proof shifts to those who deny causal relationship.

Stage 4. Government action and legislation.

Of the five examples I have chosen to study, it will be evident that cigarettes, asbestos, and some aspects of air pollution have reached stage 4; hazards from EMF are between stages 1 and 2; and lead has reached stage 3 in some countries. This panorama of five prominent public health concerns over the past forty years leads to some conclusions, as follows.

Central Role of Environmental Epidemiology

It is apparent that epidemiological studies have been central to the detection and evaluation of all these hazards. The discipline has grown (but not kept pace with) the much more general dispersion of the hazards than formerly, and with the growing realization that, the control of bacterial disease in large part attained, environmental factors underlie much human disease. Yet the fraction of research expenditure currently dedicated to epidemiological research is a very small component of the total medical research effort. The scientific community currently gives far greater emphasis to research on mechanisms of disease than to uncovering the community impact. Indeed, epidemiologists have something of the same relationship to basic medical scientists as psychiatrists have to surgeons. One hears people speak as if the basic "risk" was uncovered by animal experiments first, and then the epidemiological studies became necessary to see if the same effect was occurring in humans. In all the examples I am discussing, the epidemiological evidence preceded animal studies. Reviewing this question, Omenn (108) recently wrote:

> In conclusion, good public policy making about health risks depends on epidemiologic studies, probably more than most epidemiologists realize. Epidemiologists and toxicologists need to work at finding more common ground and more paths for integrating information from each other's field. Epidemiologists need to develop guidelines for undertaking studies or declining to do so, and epidemiologists and risk analysts need to seek convergence on terminology and descriptive language for communicating results from epidemiologic studies.

It seems proper therefore to urge that much more potential should be devoted to training and project funding in environmental epidemiology. Science awards no Nobel prizes to epidemiologists, perhaps considering that the scientific component in epidemiology is too limited.

Role of Industry and Government

It is clear that, if public health protection were to be solely dependent on dialogue between industry and government (particularly if conducted in private), the health of the public would not be protected. The lesson of eastern Europe is that government and government-controlled industry in a closed society can very easily result in a grossly degraded environment. In a free society, private collusion between industry and government (if that were the sole forum for discussion) would be likely to have the same effect.

Effective public health protection in a free society ultimately depends on legislative action. In the case of cigarettes, government intervention has shown itself to be an effective (though perhaps rather slow) mechanism for public education and persuasion to change habits and lifestyles. The U.S. Surgeon General's initiative in 1963 marked the start of a slow rollback in cigarette consumption. Without that initiative, it seems unlikely that this decline would have occurred. Similar initiatives in relation to air pollution, lead in gasoline, and the use of asbestos were central to a reduction in risks from these sources.

Much attention has recently been directed at ethical questions involving individual scientists or groups of scientists or institutions in which they work. This is perfectly proper. However, little attention has so far been directed—and perhaps it should be—at ethical constraints that should be recognized as applying to industrial consortia.

Role of Legislators (Individual and Collective)

In all jurisdictions, and in all instances, individual legislators can be identified who have spearheaded the introduction of legislation to control these hazards. Their role is therefore central. It follows that individual scientists have the responsibility of providing information, both when requested and on their own initiative, to legislators with an interest in the topics under discussion. In a free society, this is a potent resource, and one likely to result in useful initiatives. In my experience, it seems to work as well in the parliamentary system as under the United States Constitution.

Role of Public Societies and Advocacy Groups

In some instances, these have been an important component in decision-making. But the example of lead shows that effective action can be initiated and carried into legislation without a strong public advocacy group. If legislators are influenced by testimony from reputable individual and independent scientists, they can come to believe in the importance of the question in spite of strong industrial advocacy in the other direction. Where public societies exist, individual scientists have the responsibility of educating them on the problems and of ensuring that indefensible exaggeration does not occur. This is the temptation to which public advocacy groups very easily succumb. The need to maintain public subscriptions no doubt exerts pressure on such groups to push the interpretation of data beyond reasonable limits.

In spite of this limitation, one may fairly conclude that, in a free society, the existence of an informed public opinion is very important for the protection of public health. The pressures on government exerted by powerful industry are so great that, unless there is some countervailing force, the needs of public health are very unlikely to receive the priority that the public expects they should be accorded. In this context, the shift in emphasis detected by Curtis Moore (104) between the philosophy behind the U.S. Clean Air Act of 1970 and the 1990 amendments suggests that this countervailing force is more necessary now than it was twenty years ago.

Role of the Media in a Free Society

It is apparent that the media play an essential role in drawing attention to health hazards and in urging government to take some action. In spite of all the limitations in the perceptions of the media, environmental scientists and public health officials in a free society must be reconciled to the fact that they must work through and with the media. They should, I believe, undergo some instruction and guidance in relation to their future contacts with the media, and, as I have indicated, be prepared in advance for some situations. University departments that train students in environmental health issues should recognize their responsibility in relation to this question.

Role of the Independent Scientist

The central role of the independent scientist (who does not earn his or her living by representing a vested interest) is self-evident. This is why universities must be independent of the outside influence of powerful industrial consortia (acting through industrialists on boards of governors). Often, the scientists will, as I have noted earlier, feel as if they are in a "no-man's land" between warring factions, each possessed of heavy artillery. Nevertheless, the scientist must understand the difference between scientific evaluation and value judgment, and of the probability that a loose word will be taken out of context and "used against him" by one side or the other. We could probably do a more thorough job of educating young epidemiologists on these questions. Salter's (58) recent observations on scientists and advocacy would be a good place to start.

The environmental scientist may occasionally be confronted by difficult ethical questions. Merrill Eisenbud, from whose autobiography (107) I learned a great deal, gives an interesting example of this. When radioactive contamination of the Japanese fishing boat the *Lucky Dragon* (*Fukuryu Maru*) occurred after the BRAVO nuclear test in the Pacific in March 1954, he was sent at short notice by the United States government to Japan to assess the issue and consult with Japanese authorities. He was in the process of doing this when, back in the United States, President Eisenhower, accompanied by Admiral Strauss, chair of the Atomic Energy Commission, gave a televised press conference at which he said that the boat had been well within the danger area (contrary to instructions), and that the skin lesions on the fishermen "are believed to be due to the chemical activity of the converted material in the coral, rather than to radioactivity." Eisenbud knew that neither of the president's statements was true. It is perhaps surprising that Eisenbud does not discuss in detail the moral dilemma that he confronted when this occurred. Few of us are placed in such a delicate position, but we may have encountered instances in which organizations with which we were linked took actions or issued statements with which we disagreed. It may be difficult to decide whether to remonstrate in private or in public when this occurs.

Role of the Courts and the Legal Process

It is unquestionable that there are some aspects of the legal process in a free society that facilitate the often tortuous process of arriving at some decision on difficult questions. It is a strength of the legal process that eventually a decision is required. Furthermore, all the evidence has to be on the table, and the proceedings, particularly of cross-examination, have to be in the public domain.

As already noted, a disadvantage of the legal process is the common attempt to discredit a witness on grounds entirely different from the validity of his or her testimony. In the case of asbestos litigation in

the United States, so high have the financial stakes become that the
legal process has interfered with the normal components of scientific
debate. As the National Academy of Sciences has recently noted (61)
in the case of hazardous waste site litigation, adversarial counsels
may even finance quasi-epidemiological studies; they are, of course,
free not to reveal "inappropriate" conclusions. It is a current weakness of the present system in the United States that, if in such cases an
out-of-court settlement is reached, the court may order that all papers
should be sealed, and hence data from epidemiological studies relevant to public health may never be revealed.

It is a unique aspect of the United States system that a court may
have to decide whether an agency, such as the Occupational Safety
and Health Administration or the Environmental Protection Agency,
has or has not set an appropriate standard for worker or public protection. This has the effect of ensuring that the agency has examined all
of the scientific evidence, and that its assessment of risk is appropriate. Without any possibility of court action (as in the parliamentary
system), the standard-setting process within an agency may be very
casual and incomplete, and may omit the involvement of those with a
legitimate interest in the outcome. This is discussed further in the
next paragraph.

The Process of Standard Setting

I have published some thoughts on the standard-setting process elsewhere (109). The process of setting air pollution standards in the
United States involves the following steps.

1. Preparation of a criteria document. This reviews all available
scientific evidence on the matter, but does not recommend any particular number as a possible standard.

2. Approval of this document (as being comprehensive and balanced) by the Clean Air Scientific Advisory Committee of the EPA.
This has a rotating membership and consists of scientists familiar with
the field but independent of the agency. Its proceedings are publicly
available documents, and often make interesting reading.

3. Review of the criteria document by a nontechnical committee,
which sends forward specific advice (as a staff paper) to the administrator of the EPA. This committee may draw attention to particular
aspects of the criteria document, or extend its range to highlight areas

of uncertainty or to include calculations of risk for sensitive subgroups of the population.

4. The EPA administrator makes a decision; he or she usually makes it clear to what extent the proposed standard is driven by purely medical or scientific considerations, and to what extent it has had to be modified in the light of economic or other factors. A court challenge can be mounted (by the American Lung Association, or the automobile or petroleum industries for example) on the basis that the proposed standard is too lax or unnecessarily stringent.

It is in the preparation of the criteria document that problems in interpretation of data are thrashed out. Having commissioned the writing of the basic document, EPA brings together the authors, officials from the EPA office responsible for criteria documents, technical representatives of industry and environmental groups, and others. A line-by-line analysis of the document occurs. In this process, there will be detailed discussion of statistical aspects of studies, or of their design. It is because this process is so thorough (though expensive) and because all of the proceedings are in the public domain that the criteria documents are uniquely useful. Cheaper alternatives in standard setting include the convening of bureaucrats in closed session to advise on standards (as in Canada); the convening of a small group of "experts" who have forty-eight hours to agree on a figure, and then buttress their opinion with a few selected references (the procedure apparently followed by the World Health Organization); or some modification of these approaches. In the case of cancer-causing substances, a very rigorous procedure exists in Germany and has for a hundred years. A permanent board makes recommendations, but most of its members are designated by outside scientific and academic organizations; that is, the government does not control the membership. This system works well, and provides some of the advantages of other methods.

In table 2.5, the progressive tightening of the asbestos standard over a forty-year period is shown. This trend is not unique to asbestos, and has also occurred in the case of lead. Bailar (110) commented in 1989:

> The last point . . . which I call the creeping center of the information base, refers to the fact that increasing information about some hazard is much more likely to show that it is

bigger than we thought than to show it is smaller. . . . This is illustrated by some unpublished work I did in 1982 with my colleagues Judy Jackson and Emmet Keeler. We tracked the individual exposure recommendations published each year by the American Council of Governmental Industrial Hygienists (ACGIH), a private non-profit group of experts from government, academic, and research institutions, and private industry. These standards are sometimes changed, and reasons for the changes are usually given. We found that the ACGIH had published standards for 554 chemicals. Most of these were recently published, with little time for possible revisions, but 175 standards had been changed a total of 222 times. Of these, 185 changes, or 83%, were in the direction of reducing allowable exposures. Of these 222 changes, 114 were on the basis of new evidence (33 animal studies, 81 human studies), 46 were on the basis of new interpretations of old evidence, and 35 seemed to be from concern that margins of safety were too small; we could not classify 27 changes. The conclusion seems inescapable that, at least in the experience in the United States, exposure limits tend to become tighter with time, and these changes are driven largely by increases in scientific information. It would seem good public policy to recognize this tendency and to set initial exposure limits somewhat lower than present evidence justifies.

Unfortunately, it seems unlikely that this good advice will be heeded. It may be objected that few standards have ever been relaxed because it would not be worth the effort to go through a process to change them, even though new scientific evidence may show that the risk is less than previously indicated.

I conclude from this brief consideration of the role of the standard-setting process that it can provide and has provided a uniquely useful mechanism for considering the strength of all the evidence that bears on the process of protecting the public health. The discussion of the detailed data—whether they are epidemiological or experimental, in a nonjudicial but public forum in which the temptation to score points by character denigration is absent—can lead to a very productive dialogue. The need to try to reconcile conflicting data, if such exist, and to concentrate attention on the final object of the discussion—namely, to be able to reach consensus on some definitive number as a minimal effects level for example—together have the effect of focusing the discussion in a manner that would not otherwise exist.

Such deliberations should occur within a diverse group. If a specific group of workers are at special risk, as they may be from such hazards as asbestos or radon, their representatives should participate in the discussion (111). The placing of the proceedings in the public domain acts to prevent too partisan a point of view.

This process of arriving at a consensus on a safe standard for public exposure could be structured as a "consensus conference" of the type visualized by Wessel (106). A government agency or ministry could well finance a process of this kind, without necessarily being bound by the outcome, and by so doing encourage a convergence of views. I have observed that this kind of mechanism is only feared by those who suspect (rightly) that they cannot control the outcome.

I have noted that the British have often in the past been reluctant to agree to the propounding of any standard for maximal permitted exposure to anything, usually arguing that the scientific data are not strong enough for any conclusion to be reached. Other countries, particularly the United States and some European countries, have taken the view that a standard is always necessary if the public health is to be protected. Canada has oscillated between these two viewpoints, often being content to publish "guidelines"; these are relatively weak because they do not require specific action when they are transgressed.

The Role of Consensus Conferences

Wessel (106) argued the value of conferences designed to produce a consensus on a question. Another mechanism is to establish an interdisciplinary committee, give it enough time to work, and require it to produce a report that represents a consensus of members. This is what the special advisory committee to the EPA's Science Advisory Board (74) was required to do (with the additional requirement that its deliberations should be in public). Governments can facilitate this process when the need is perceived. In the United States system, hearings before special committees of the Senate play a very important role; unfortunately there is no effective and equivalent process in the parliamentary system. However, the conference committees that operate in the United States to negotiate a compromise between the House of Representatives and the Senate do not do so in public. In the parliamentary system, on some occasions, committees have been constituted with members from the different parties in the House of Commons. This was done in the case of proposed cigarette legislation, and in connection with the problem of acid rain. These committees may suffer from lack of a strong, permanent, and well-informed staff, and usually either produce recommendations that are never implemented (as was the case in Canada in relation to an inter-parliamentary committee on cigarettes), or their proceedings degenerate into party political squabbling.

The production of "objective" reports steered by organizations that are perceived to be independent of interested parties (such as the Health Effects Institute [47]) provides another mechanism. However the disadvantage here is that there is no opportunity for public input and no dialogue, therefore, in relation to the most difficult questions. There is, after all, a great deal to be said for the process of cross-examination; particularly is this the case in clarifying the basis of different opinions on the interpretation of epidemiological data. Only in this way can the (unstated) value assumptions that necessarily underlie such opinions be brought out into the open.

Differences Between the Parliamentary System and the United States Constitution

Several major differences between political processes in the parliamentary system, as seen in Britain and in Canada, and the United States system affect decision-making processes on environmental questions. In a parliamentary country, accountability is attained by such traditions as "question time" in the House of Commons; the election process provides an opportunity to defeat a government with unpopular policies. Actual power is exerted by the cabinet. All ministers are elected politicians. Challenges to government action—such as that forbidding the use of saccharin, the spraying of asbestos, or the use of lead in gasoline—can only be mounted on the basis that a minister has exceeded the power vested in him or her. No legal challenge is possible on the basis that the scientific data have been misread or disregarded. Ministers in the parliamentary system may (and do) appoint advisory committees to themselves that may report confidentially. Under the Public Inquiry Act, the federal or a provincial government may appoint a royal commission required to have public input and to report in public. This inquiry system has been commonly used in Canada, and the process has been the subject of considerable study (112). Apart from such inquiries, the parliamentary system encourages a closed decision-making process, but action to deal with a problem (such as a hazardous waste site) can be very swift and unchallengeable.

In the United States, the decision that, if a citizen wished to challenge an action by a government agent, he should have recourse to a court process, was taken by its first president, George Washington (113). The question involved "an aggrieved owner of a carriage who asserted an incorrect classification of his pleasure vehicle by the internal revenue agent." Carriages were apparently taxed on the basis of their wheelbases. In deciding that a court should arbitrate between a citizen and a government representative, Washington was no doubt reacting to the arbitrary exercise of government power that characterized the British government of that era. His decision has had profound repercussions. Today, for example, it means that the American Petroleum Institute can mount a court challenge to a proposed air pollution standard; because of this possibility, the process of deciding on the standard has to be much more rigorous. This process of court challenge lay dormant until about 1965, but it has been increasingly used since then. The administrator in charge of the Environmental Protection Agency (who is about to become a member of the cabinet) is not an elected official but an appointed one approved by the U.S. Senate. Decisions on environmental action are therefore one step removed from the direct two-party system, though in effect no important action can be taken without the concurrence of the White House. The influence of the president, and particularly of his advisers, is considerable in determining which agenda items are pushed and which relegated to the back burner.

The strength of the United States system lies in the power vested in committees of Congress. All the major discussion that preceded the original Clean Air Act, and its more recent successor, took place in public before a Senate committee. Senators are given sufficient resources to employ specialized staff. In my experience, their knowledge of the technicalities of air pollution and its control is prodigious, and generally not matched by deputy ministers in the parliamentary system. Political horse-trading in relation to decisions affecting public health and the environment undoubtedly occurs and will presumably occur in the future, but the final decisions are backed by formidable technical expertise. An act passed in the United States in 1970 expressly forbade agencies to receive from advisory committees reports that remained confidential, except in certain defined circumstances.

Those operating within the parliamentary system tend to ridicule the dominant role of lawyers in the United States process, but concede that the process is a much more open one; those in the United States marvel at the closed decision-making process still customary in the parliamentary system, but envy the ability of the system to take swift and unchallenged action.

Offsetting Public Disenchantment with the Process of Decision Making

Anyone who has listened to a large volume of public input on a contentious question involving public health comes to realize that a significant segment of society views the world only in terms of conspiracy theories, believing that industry, government, and individual scientists constitute a formidable cabal seeking to deny the validity of epidemiological data and to discredit anyone who expresses a contrary opinion. The recent volume on the adverse health effects of electromagnetic fields (80) is written from this standpoint. An extension of such a view is to regard all information as subjective, to deny that any objective data can exist, and hence to treat all phenomena as if they were the result of "magic." Salter (58) notes the basis for the contemporary disenchantment of society with scientists—they can, after all, be bought like anything else.

It is important to stress a contrary view of the world. It is necessary to assert that it is possible to establish whether lead in low doses affects the development of children, and if so, how. It is possible to do research to form a judgment on whether current levels of air pollution are injurious. It is necessary to maintain on all occasions that we do know something about how to establish objectively reliable information; and that correct answers to questions of fact do actually exist. Such an assertion will never convince a small minority of the public, but that is what they are, a small minority.

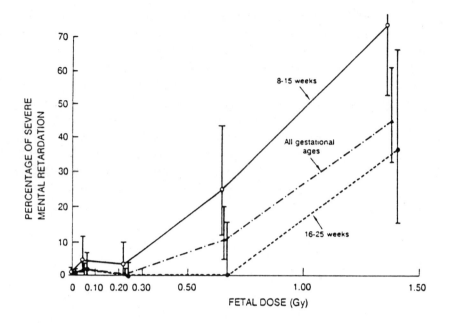

Figure 5.1. Percentage of severe mental retardation among those exposed in utero by dose and gestational age in Hiroshima and Nagasaki. Vertical lines indicate 90 percent confidence intervals. Source: NRC (1990). From reference 114. These recently published data from the Hiroshima and Nagasaki exposed population are a chilling reminder of the vulnerability of the developing brain. It is remarkable that they have attracted (so far) very little media attention.

Respect for the Complexity of Living Processes

Albert Schweitzer taught "reverence for life" as an important philosophical and ethical attitude. Reviewing the five hazards I have chosen to discuss, I am made aware of two entirely disparate attitudes. On the one hand, I see a mystical approach to life and living, which, in extreme form, seeks to deny the validity of any scientific evidence; and on the other, perhaps exemplified by engineers (48), I observe a mechanistic (and simplistic) approach to biological outcomes. This is another "no-man's land" in which the independent environmental scientist may well find himself.

We can at the very least, I suggest, stress the complexity of living processes. The public is surely right in believing that our entrepreneurial ingenuity in introducing new chemicals or new processes into our environment, and disseminating them widely, far outstrips our ability to assess them. Furthermore, our understanding of such extraordinarily complex processes as the growth and development of the human brain is still so rudimentary that foresight can hardly be required of us. A chilling reminder of the reality of this is shown in figure 5.1. I began by recalling the 1945 bombing of Hiroshima and Nagasaki; this figure shows data published only a year ago indicating that the in utero radiation that resulted from those events led to a major (and dose-response related) increase in severe mental retardation.

What is currently required of us is undoubtedly to stress the limitations of our biological understanding, and to counter an attitude of "environmental bravado" whenever we detect it, for it is surely based on ignorance.

We should have learned enough over the past forty years to know that such an attitude is a sure recipe for disaster.

References

1. Corn, J. K., and Starr, J. 1987. Historical perspective on asbestos: policies and protective measures in World War II shipbuilding. *American Journal of Industrial Medicine* 11:359–373.
2. Lippmann, M. 1992. Ozone. In *Environmental toxicants: human exposures and their health effects,* ed. Morton Lippmann. New York: Van Nostrand Reinhold.
3. Thompson, J. 1991. East Europe's dark dawn. *National Geographic* 179: 36–39.
4. Leowski, J. 1986. Mortality from acute respiratory infections in children under 5 years of age; global estimates. *World Health Statistics Quarterly* 39:138–144.
5. Pandey, M. R., Smith, K. R., Boleij, J. S. M., and Wafula, E. M. 1989. Indoor air pollution in developing countries and acute respiratory infection in children. *Lancet* (25 February):427–429.
6. Cohen, N. 1991. Regulation of in-place asbestos-containing material. *Environmental Research* 55:97–106.
7. Bates, D. V. 1972. *A citizen's guide to air pollution.* Montreal and London: McGill-Queen's University Press.
8. Rose, G. 1989. Science, ethics and public policy. In *Assessment of health hazards,* ed. U. Mohr, pp. 349–356. Heidelberg and New York: Springer-Verlag.
9. The effects of fog on cattle in London. *The Veterinarian* XLVII:533 (Fourth Series no. 299), January 1874.
10. Seiberling, G. 1988. *Monet in London.* Seattle and London: University of Washington Press.
11. H. M. Stationery Office. 1954. *Mortality and morbidity during the London fog of December 1952.* Report no. 95 on Public Health and Medical Subjects. London.

12. Ashby, E., and Anderson, M. 1981. *The politics of clean air.* Oxford: Clarendon Press.

13. Tarr, J. A. 1981. Changing fuel use behavior and energy transitions: the Pittsburgh smoke control movement 1940–1950. *Journal of Social History* 14:561–588.

14. Royal College of Physicians. 1970. *Air pollution and health: a report for the Royal College of Physicians.* London: Pitman Medical and Scientific Publishing Co.

15. Haagen-Smit, A. J. 1952. Chemistry and physiology of Los Angeles smog. *Industrial and Engineering Chemistry* 44:1342–1346.

16. Holland, W. W., and Reid, D. D. 1965. The urban factor in chronic bronchitis. *Lancet* 1:445–48.

17. Xu, X., Dockery, D. W., and Wang, L. 1991. Effects of air pollution on adult pulmonary function. *Archives of Environmental Health* 46:198–206.

18. Bates, D. V. 1994. The effects of photochemical air pollution on people. In *Tropospheric ozone: human health and agricultural impacts,* ed. David J. McKee. Boca Raton: Lewis Publishers.

19. Koren, H. S., Devlin, R. B., Graham, D. E., Man, R., McGee, M. P., Horstman, D. H., Kozumbo, W. J., Becker, S., House, D. E., McDonnell, W. F., and Bromberg, P. A. 1869. Ozone-induced inflammation in the lower airways of human subjects. *American Review of Respiratory Diseases* 139:407–415.

20. Hazucha, M., Bates, D. V., and Bromberg, P. A. 1989. Mechanism of action of ozone on the human lung. *Journal of Applied Physiology* 67:1535–1541.

21. Kreit, J. W., Gross, K. B., Moore, T. B., Lorenzen, T. J., D'Arcy, J., and Eschenbacher, W. L. 1989. Ozone-induced changes in pulmonary function and bronchial responsiveness in asthmatics. *Journal of Applied Physiology* 66:217–222.

22. Keeler, G. J., Spengler, J. D., Koutrakis, P., Allen, G. A., Raizenne, M., and Stern, B. 1990. Transported acid aerosols measured in southern Ontario. *Atmospheric Environment* 24A:2935–2950.

23. Bates, D. V., and Sizto, R. 1987. Hospital admissions and air pollutants in southern Ontario: the acid summer haze effect. *Environmental Research* 43:317–331.

24. Bates, D. V. 1985. The strength of the evidence relating air pollutants to adverse health effects. Carolina Environmental Essay Series. Chapel Hill: University of North Carolina Institute for Environmental Studies.

25. Thurston, G. D., Ito, K., Lippmann, M., and Bates, D. V. In press. Respiratory hospital admissions and summertime haze air pollution in Toronto, Ontario: consideration of the role of acid aerosols.

26. Schwartz, J., and Dockery, D. W. 1992. Increased mortality in Philadelphia associated with daily air pollution concentrations. *American Review of Respiratory Diseases* 145:600–604.

27. Sebastian, I. 1990. Issues in urban air pollution: Ankara diagnostic report. Environment Working Paper, no. 38. Washington, D.C.: World Bank.

28. Warner, K. E. 1989. Effects of the antismoking campaign: an update. *American Journal of Public Health* 79:144–151.

29. Ritchie, J. W., 1930. *Human Physiology*. Rev. W. J. Dobbie. Canadian Health Series. Toronto: W. J. Gage & Co., Ltd.

30. Gould, S. J. 1991. The smoking gun of eugenics. *Natural History* 12:9–17.

31. U.S. National Academy of Sciences. 1986. Environmental tobacco smoke. Washington, D.C.: National Academy Press.

32. U.S. Department of Health and Human Services. 1986. *The health consequences of involuntary smoking*. Washington, D.C.

33. Samet, J.M. 1989. Environmental tobacco smoke: adverse effects on respiratory infection, respiratory symptoms, and lung function. In *Assessment of inhalational hazards*, ed. U. Mohr. Heidelberg and New York: Springer-Verlag.

34. Lee, P. N., Fry, J. S., and Forey, B. A. 1990. Trends in lung cancer, chronic obstructive lung disease, and emphysema death rates for England and Wales 1941–1985 and their relation to trends in cigarette smoking. *Thorax* 45:657–665.

35. Snider, G. L. 1992. Emphysema: the first two centuries—and beyond: a historical overview, with suggestions for future research; part I. *American Review of Respiratory Diseases* 146:1334–1344.

36. Fielding, J. E. 1987. Smoking and women. *New England Journal of Medicine* 317:1343–1345.

37. Fielding, J. E. 1985. Smoking: health effects and control. *New England Journal of Medicine* 313:491–498.

38. Doll, R. 1983. Prospects for prevention. *British Medical Journal* 286:445–453.

39. Warner, K. E. 1989. Effects of the antismoking campaign: an update. *American Journal of Public Health* 79:144–151.

40. Pierce, J. P. 1989. International comparisons of trends in cigarette smoking prevalence. *American Journal of Public Health* 79:152–157.

41. Pierce, J. P. 1991. Progress and problems in international public health efforts to reduce tobacco usage. *Annual Review of Public Health* 12:383–400.

42. Mancuso, T. F. 1989. Letter to the editor: response to Dr. C-G Ohlson. *American Journal of Industrial Medicine* 15:353–356.

43. Becklake, M. R. 1976. Asbestos-related diseases of the lung and other organs: their epidemiology and implications for clinical practice. *American Review of Respiratory Diseases* 114:187–227.

44. International Agency for Research on Cancer. 1973. *Biological effects of asbestos; proceedings of a working conference, October 2–6, 1972*. Lyon, France.

45. Brodeur, P. 1985. *Outrageous misconduct: the asbestos industry on trial*. New York: Pantheon Books.

46. Lippmann, M. 1992. Asbestos and other mineral fibers. In *Environmental toxicants: human exposures and their health effects*, ed. Morton Lippmann. New York: Van Nostrand Reinhold.

47. Health Effects Institute. 1991. *Asbestos in public and commercial buildings: a literature review and synthesis of current knowledge*. Cambridge, Mass.

48. Bates, D. V. 1991. Editorial: asbestos—the turbulent interface between science and policy. *Canadian Medical Association Journal* 144:554–556.
49. Henneberger, P. K., and Stanbury, M. J. 1992. Patterns of asbestosis in New Jersey. *American Journal of Industrial Medicine* 21:689–697.
50. Burdorf, L., Swuste, P. H. J. J., and Heederik, D. 1991. A history of awareness of asbestos disease and the control of occupational asbestos exposures in the Netherlands. *American Journal of Industrial Medicine* 20:547–555.
51. Shepherd, K. E., Oliver, L. C., and Kazemi, H. 1989. Diffuse malignant pleural mesothelioma in an urban hospital: clinical spectrum and trend in incidence over time. *American Journal of Industrial Medicine* 16:373–383.
52. Huncharek, M. 1992. Changing risk groups for malignant mesothelioma. *Cancer* 69:2704–2711.
53. Churg, A., Wright, J. L., Gilks, B., and Depaoli, L. 1989. Rapid short-term clearance of chrysotile compared with amosite asbestos in the guinea pig. *American Review of Respiratory Diseases* 139:885–890.
54. Du Toit, R. S. J. 1991. An estimate at which crocidolite asbestos fibres are cleared from the lung. *Annals of Occupational Hygiene* 35:433–438.
55. Churg, A., and Wiggs, B. 1986. Fiber size and number in users of processed chrysotile ore, chrysotile miners, and members of the general population. *American Journal of Industrial Medicine* 9:143–152.
56. Churg, A. 1991. Editorial: analysis of lung asbestos content. *British Journal of Industrial Medicine* 48:649–652.
57. Bates, D. V. 1987. Editorial: asbestos; promotion or prohibition? *Canadian Medical Association Journal* 26:107–109.
58. Salter, L. 1988. *Mandated science: science and scientists in the making of standards.* Dordrecht, Boston, and London: Kluwer Academic Publishers.
59. Hertzman, C., Ward, H., Ames, N., Kelly, S., and Yates, C. 1991. Childhood lead exposure in Trail revisited. *Canadian Journal of Public Health* 82:385–391.
60. Mahaffey, K. E. R., McKinney, J., and Reigart, J. R. 1992. Lead and compounds. In *Environmental toxicants: human exposures and their health effects,* ed. Morton Lippmann. New York: Van Nostrand Reinhold.
61. U.S. National Academy of Science. 1992. *Environmental epidemiology; Vol 2.: data gaps, resource needs and research opportunities.* Washington, D.C.
62. Needleman, H. L., and Gatsonis, C. A. 1990. Low-level lead exposure and the IQ of children: a meta-analysis of modern studies. *Journal of the American Medical Association* 263:673–678.
63. Royal Society of Canada. Commission on Lead. 1986. *Lead in the Canadian environment: science and regulation; final report.* Ottawa, Ont.: Royal Society of Canada.
64. Peterson, E. B., Chan, Y-H., Peterson, N. M., Constable, G. A., Caton, R. B., Davis, C. S., Wallace, R. R., and Yarrenton, G. A. 1987. *Cumulative effects assessment in Canada: an agenda for action and research.* Ottawa, Ont.: Minister of Supply and Services, Canadian Environmental Assessment Research Council.

65. Winneke, G., Brockhaus, A., Ewers, U., Kramer, U., and Neuf, M. 1990. Results from the European multicenter study on lead neurotoxicity in children: implications for risk assessment. *Neurotoxicology and Teratology* 12:553–559.

66. Smith, M. A. 1988. *The neuropsychological effects of lead in children: a review of the research report from the Medical Research Council Advisory Group on Lead and Neuropsychological Effects in Children.* London: Hospital for Sick Children, Institute of Child Health, Department of Child Psychiatry.

67. U.S. National Academy of Sciences. 1992. *Environmental Neurotoxicology.* Washington, D.C.: National Academy Press.

68. Smith, M. A., Grant, L. D., and Sors, A. I., eds. 1988. *Lead exposure and child development: an international assessment.* Report published for the Commission of the European Communities and the U.S. Environmental Protection Agency. Dordrecht, Boston, and London: Kluwer Academic Publishers.

69. Lippmann, M. 1990. Lead and human health: background and recent findings. 1989 Alice Hamilton Lecture. *Environmental Research* 51:1–24.

70. World Health Organization. Regional Office for Europe. 1987. *Air quality guidelines for Europe.* WHO Regional Publications, European Series, no. 23. Geneva, Switzerland.

71. National Radiological Protection Board (U.K.). 1992. *Electromagnetic fields and the risk of cancer; report of an advisory group on nonionising radiation.* Vol. 3, no. 1. Chilton, England.

72. Wertheimer, N., and Leeper, E. 1979 Electrical wiring configurations and childhood cancer. *American Journal of Epidemiology* 109:273–284.

73. U.S. Environmental Protection Agency. Office of Research and Development. 1990. *Evaluation of the potential carcinogenicity of electromagnetic fields; review draft.* Washington, D.C.

74. U.S. Environmental Protection Agency. Science Advisory Board. 1991. *Potential carcinogenicity of electromagnetic fields; report of the Nonionizing Electric and Magnetic Fields Subcommittee of the Radiation Advisory Committee of the Science Advisory Board.* Washington, D.C.

75. Theriault, G. 1992. Electromagnetic fields and cancer risks. *Rev Epidem et Sante Publ* 40:S55–S62.

76. London, S. J., Thomas, D. C., Bowman, J. D., Sobel, E., Cheng, T-C., and Peters, J. M. 1991. Exposure to residential electric and magnetic fields and risk of childhood leukemia. *American Journal of Epidemiology* 134:923–937.

77. Hutchison, G. B. 1991. Carcinogenic effects of exposure to electric fields and magnetic fields. Paper prepared for Workshop on Future Epidemiologic Studies of Health Effects of Electric Fields and Magnetic Fields, Carmel, California, Feb. 6–8, 1991.

78. Feychting, M., and Ahlboom A. 1992. *Magnetic fields and cancer in people residing near Swedish high voltage power lines.* Stockholm: Karolinska Institutet, Institutet for Miljomedicin.

79. Floderus, B., Persson, T., et al. 1992. *Occupational exposure to electromagnetic fields in relation to leukemia and brain tumors; a case-control study.* Solna,

Sweden: National Institute of Occupational Health, Department of Neuromedicine.

80. Brodeur, P. 1989. *Currents of death: power lines, computer terminals, and the attempt to cover up their threat to your health.* New York: Simon and Schuster.

81. Graham, L. R. 1981. *Between science and values.* New York: Columbia University Press.

82. Steensberg, J. 1989. *Environmental health decision-making: the politics of disease prevention.* Copenhagen: Almquist and Wiksell International.

83. Stigler, S. M. 1986. *The history of statistics: the measurement of uncertainty before 1900.* Cambridge, Mass.: Belknap Press of Harvard University Press.

84. Rothman, K. J., ed. 1988. *Causal Inference.* Chestnut Hill, Mass.: Epidemiology Resources, Inc.

85. Hill, A. B. 1965. The environment and disease: association or causation? *Proceedings of the Royal Society of Medicine* 58:295–300.

86. Bates, D. V. 1992. Health indices of the adverse effects of air pollution: the question of coherence. *Environmental Research* 59:336–349.

87. Saracci, R. 1981. Personal-environmental interactions in occupational epidemiology. In *Recent advances in occupational health,* ed. J. C. McDonald. London: Churchill Livingstone.

88. Harrison, K., and Hoberg, G. In press. *Risk, science, and politics: regulating toxic substances in Canada and the United States.*

89. Checkoway, H., and Hickey, J. L. S. 1988. Estimating the potential disease rate reduction under varying conditions of combined effects. *International Journal of Epidemiology* 17:666–672.

90. Omenn, G. S., Merchant, J., Boatman, E., Dement, J. M., Kuschner, M., Nicholson, W., Peto, J., and Rosenstock, L. 1986. Contribution of environmental fibers to respiratory cancer. *Environmental Health Perspectives* 70:51–56.

91. Gould, S. J. 1992. The confusion over evolution. *New York Review of Books* 39:47–54.

92. Rose, G. 1987. Environmental factors and disease: the manmade environment. *British Medical Journal* 294:963–965.

93. Corn, J. K. 1992. *Response to occupational health hazards: a historical perspective.* New York: Van Nostrand Reinhold.

94. Rosenthal, A., Gray, G. M., and Graham, J. D. 1992. Legislating acceptable cancer risk from exposure to toxic chemicals. *Ecology Law Quarterly* 19:269–362.

95. Seixas, N. S., Robins, T. G., Attfield, M. S., and Moulton, L. H. 1992. Exposure-response relationships for coal mine dust and obstructive lung disease following enactment of the Federal Coal Mine Health and Safety Act of 1969. *American Journal of Industrial Medicine* 21:715–734.

96. Sanden, A., Jarvholm, B., Larsson, S., and Thiringer, G. 1992. The risk of lung cancer and mesothelioma after cessation of asbestos exposure: a prospective cohort study of shipyard workers. *European Respiratory Journal* 5:281–285.

97. Upton, A. C. 1992. Perspectives on individual and community risks. In *Environmental toxicants: human exposures and their health effects*, ed. Morton Lippmann. New York: Van Nostrand Reinhold.

98. Blodgett, J. 1989. *Health benefits of air pollution control: a discussion*. Congressional Research Service Report for Congress. Washington, D.C.: U.S. Library of Congress.

99. U.S. Environmental Protection Agency. Economic Analysis Division. 1985. *Costs and benefits of reducing lead in gasoline: final regulatory impact analysis*. Washington, D.C.

100. Hall, J. W., Winer, A. M., Kleinman, M. T., Lurmann, F. W., Brajer, V., and Colome, S. D. 1992. Valuing the health benefits of clean air. *Science* 255:812–817.

101. Russell, M. 1988. Ozone pollution: the hard choices. *Science* 241:1275–1276.

102. Porter, M. E. 1991. Essay: America's green strategy. *Scientific American* 264:168.

103. Moore, C. A. 1992. Bush's nonsense on jobs and the environment. *The New York Times*, September 25, 1992.

104. Moore, C. A. 1992. The 1990 Clean Air Act amendments: silk purse or sow's ear? *Duke Environmental Law and Policy Forum* 2:26–58.

105. Science Council of Canada. 1982. *Regulating the regulators: science, values and decisions*. Report no. 35. Ottawa, Ont.: Minister of Supply and Services.

106. Wessel, M. R. 1980. *Science and conscience*. New York: Columbia University Press.

107. Eisenbud, M. 1990. *An environmental odyssey: people, pollution, and politics in the life of a practical scientist*. Seattle: University of Washington Press.

108. Omenn, G. S. In press. The role of environmental epidemiology in public policy. *Annals of Epidemiology*.

109. Bates, D. V. 1988. Standard-setting as an integrative exercise: alchemy, juggling, or science? In *Inhalation toxicology*, ed. U. Mohr. Heidelberg and New York: Springer-Verlag.

110. Bailar, J. C. 1989. Inhalation hazards: the interpretation of epidemiologic evidence. In *Assessment of inhalation hazards*, ed. U. Mohr. Heidelberg and New York: Springer-Verlag.

111. Science Council of Canada. 1977. *Policies and poisons*. Report no. 28. Ottawa, Ont.

112. Salter, L., and Slaco, D. 1981. *Public enquiries in Canada*. Science Council of Canada Background Study no. 47. Ottawa, Ont.: Minister of Supply and Services.

113. White, L. D. 1948. *The Federalists: a study in administrative history 1789–1801*. New York: Free Press.

114. U.S. National Research Council. 1990. *Health effects of exposure to low levels of ionizing radiation (BIER 5)*. Washington, D.C.: National Academy Press.

Index